The Doctor's Guide to Vitamin B6

The Doctor's Guide to Vitamin B6

By
Alan
Gaby, M.D.

Rodale Press, Emmaus, Pennsylvania

Book design by Linda Jacopetti

Printed in the United States of America on recycled paper containing a high percentage of de-inked fiber.

Library of Congress Cataloging in Publication Data

Gaby, Alan.
　　The doctor's guide to vitamin B_6.

　　Includes index.
　　　1. Vitamin B_6.　　2. Vitamin B_6—Therapeutic use.
I. Title.
QP772.P9G33　　1984　　　　615'.328　　　　84-11747
ISBN 0-87857-516-2　hardcover
ISBN 0-87857-518-9　paperback
2　4　6　8　10　9　7　5　3　1　hardcover
2　4　6　8　10　9　7　5　3　1　paperback

To my parents and to Erica for caring and understanding.

Notice

The information and ideas in this book are for educational purposes and must not be taken as prescriptive advice. Self-treatment can be dangerous, so check with your physician if you have a serious health problem. Also, be aware that very high doses of vitamin B_6 must not be taken. In general, you should not exceed 50 milligrams daily without medical supervision. If you are under medical care or taking medication, consult your physician before taking B_6.

Contents

A Caution

No vitamin or other healthful substance should be abused to the point where it becomes harmful. Vitamin B_6 can become toxic if taken in high doses. In general, a conservative approach would be to take no more than 50 milligrams a day unless you are otherwise advised by a knowledgeable physician. If you are under medical care or taking medication, check with your physician before taking B_6.

Acknowledgments

John M. Ellis, M.D., for making us all aware of the importance of vitamin B_6.

Jonathan Wright, M.D., for helping shape my philosophy and understanding of nutritional medicine.

William Gottlieb and Joann Williams for coordinating the writing of this book.

Jan Bresnick for her excellent and professional work of editing the manuscript.

The *Prevention* research staff—Martha Capwell, Holly Clemson, Christy Kohler, Carol Pribulka, Carole Rapp, Nancy Smerkanich and Susan Zarrow—for carefully checking the accuracy of my statements and references.

Eve Perlberg and Samuel D. Gaby, M.D., for their painstaking proofreading.

And thanks to Diana Gottshall and Susan Lagler.

Part B₆:I

Part

B₆:I
Our Changing
Requirement

Chapter

How Much Do We Need? 1

Until recently, vitamin B_6 was considered something of a "second-line" vitamin, not worthy of the status accorded to thiamine (vitamin B_1), niacinamide (vitamin B_3), vitamin B_{12} or ascorbic acid (vitamin C). Lack of thiamine was known to cause beriberi, a serious and sometimes fatal disease. Niacinamide deficiency caused pellagra (dementia, dermatitis, diarrhea and death). Low levels of vitamins C and B_{12} led to scurvy and pernicious anemia, respectively. Unlike these nutrients, B_6 had not yet been associated with a specific nutritional deficiency disease, and there was little evidence that pyridoxine (B_6) deficiency posed any great risk for the average person.

In the past decade, our thinking about vitamin B_6 has changed dramatically. From relative obscurity this vitamin has emerged as one of the most talked about nutrients. Dozens of reports in the medical literature have demonstrated the value of B_6 supplements for a wide range of problems.

In 1973 P. W. Adams, M.D., and co-workers discovered that B_6 supplements would often relieve the emotional depression that develops in some women who take birth control pills. The same year, John M. Ellis, M.D., reported on his successful use of B_6 as a remedy for the "carpal tunnel syndrome," a nerve compression syndrome that causes numbness, pain and weakness in the hands.

In 1975 Platon J. Collipp, M.D., and associates reported in the *Annals of Allergy* that B_6 supplements helped some children suffering from asthma. Two years later, David Byar, M.D., and Clyde Blackard, M.D., presented evidence that vitamin B_6 might help prevent recurrences of bladder cancer. In 1978 the *American Journal of Podiatry* featured a report that B_6 had eliminated the numbness, burning, tingling, joint pains and swelling that occurs in the legs and feet of some diabetics. Around the same time, Robert A. Rojer, M.D., and associates found that B_6 supplements dramatically improved the anemia that occurs in a blood disorder called primary myelofibrosis.

In 1979 Mary Coleman, M.D., published a paper showing that B_6 relieved symptoms and calmed the behavior of some hyperactive children. The following year Guy E. Abraham, M.D., and Joel T. Hargrove, M.D., demonstrated that B_6 is an effective treatment for most women suffering from moderate or severe premenstrual tension and swelling, and apparently restored fertility in some previously infertile women. In 1981 Karl Folkers, Ph.D., and colleagues determined that vitamin B_6 supplements may prevent the uncomfortable symptoms of Chinese restaurant syndrome. That same year, an editorial appearing in the respected medical journal *Lancet* concluded that additional B_6 might help prevent heart disease.

In 1983 Claes Hallert, M.D., reported on his successful use of B_6 as a treatment for mental depression associated with celiac disease. Other studies during the past decade have demonstrated that B_6 may help prevent kidney stones, improve the functioning of autistic children and relieve the psychological depression that often accompanies chronic kidney failure.

The effectiveness and versatility of this interesting vitamin are certainly impressive, if not entirely surprising. Vitamin B_6 is, you see, one of the most heavily worked coenzymes, a group of small molecules that act as keys, turning on and off most biochemical reactions.

As recently as 1970, B_6 wasn't considered particularly useful. Sure, there were a few rare genetic diseases known to respond to this vitamin, and it was occasionally used to prevent the toxic effects of certain drugs. A minority of doctors believed that B_6 relieved nausea and vomiting of pregnancy. Several other reports that appeared over the years suggested a minor therapeutic role for vitamin B_6. But until the 1970's, no one seemed to be aware of B_6's value in such a wide range of common medical conditions.

Why is it that vitamin B_6, nearly half a century after its discovery, has suddenly developed such exciting therapeutic potential? The obvious explanation is that modern scientists, with their sophisticated research equipment and insightful minds, have been able to discover things their predecessors had overlooked. In other words, B_6 has always been valuable; it's just that very few people realized it. Although this explanation seems simple enough, it's probably not correct.

On the contrary, scientists of yesteryear were a lot more aware than "modern science chauvinists" would have us believe. They were shrewd observers with fertile minds. They were aware of many nutritional phenomena that are only now being rediscovered. For example, it had been suggested as early as 1944 (about 25 years before Linus Pauling revived the idea) that vitamin C might be able to reduce the severity of colds and influenza.[1] Exciting new research showing that essential fatty acids improve eczema is not really new at all—doctors had discovered that in 1933.[2] Likewise, modern research on the anticancer effect of vitamin A can be traced back as far as 1932.[3] Some doctors were advocating allergy-elimination diets to treat migraine headaches 60 years before this method was popularized by the current generation of medical nutritionists. Our predecessors in the field discovered countless other nutritional pearls that are only now coming back into vogue. But about vitamin B_6 there was hardly a word.

A New Deficiency

If we accept that scientists working prior to World War II were good at what they did, it seems unlikely that they would have been unaware of how valuable B_6 is. I believe there's another reason for B_6's recent usefulness: Widespread deficiency is a new problem.

This proposition is not as farfetched as you might think. Consider that some of the diseases that respond to B_6 have become much more common. It stands to reason that B_6 deficiency might be on the rise as well. In other words, people seem to need far more of this vitamin today than in previous generations. We may be witnessing a virtual epidemic of B_6 deficiency.

Carpal tunnel syndrome—caused by pressure on the median nerve as it passes down the arm, through a structure in the wrist called the carpal tunnel, and into the hand—is a prime example of this epidemic. Vitamin B_6 somehow relieves this nerve pressure and the symptoms that go with it. Carpal tunnel syndrome is now encountered quite frequently by the average physician, although as recently as 1950 it seems to have been a relatively rare problem. In that year George Phalen, M.D., a pioneer in the surgical treatment of carpal tunnel syndrome, presented his first 11 cases at the 99th annual meeting of the American

Medical Association. Dr. Phalen noted that very few physicians at that meeting were familiar with the syndrome he described,[4] but in the 30 years since, carpal tunnel syndrome has become widespread.

Other diseases associated with a need for extra B_6 have also become more prevalent. The incidence of kidney stones has doubled in the United States and Great Britain since the 1960's.[5] Attention deficit disorder (hyperactivity) was not viewed as a widespread problem until the 1970's. Today an estimated 5 to 20 percent of all children in this country suffer from some form of attention deficit. Premenstrual syndrome (PMS), also effectively treated with vitamin B_6, is now said to affect between 70 and 90 percent of all American women. Until recently, little was written about it in the medical literature. While social factors have definitely contributed to an increased awareness of premenstrual syndrome, it seems likely that the true incidence has also increased. All this circumstantial evidence suggests that the need for more vitamin B_6 is a new problem, and a rather frequent one at that.

What has happened in the past few decades that could have touched off this epidemic of B_6 deficiency? Is our steady consumption of refined sugar, white flour and overprocessed food the culprit? An analysis of our modern food supply shows that many of us are consuming less than the Recommended Dietary Allowance (RDA) for vitamin B_6.[6] On the other hand, a sugar-laden, nutrient-depleted diet has been with us for quite some time. If we are consuming less B_6 than we did 50 years ago, the difference couldn't amount to more than a few tenths of a milligram a day.

Could such a small change in the dietary level of B_6 be the straw that broke the camel's back, plunging millions of us into a state of deficiency? That is an unlikely explanation, because the new epidemic of B_6 deficiency appears to be more than just a dietary shortage. The RDA for vitamin B_6 is only about 2 milligrams a day. If all we were doing with B_6 therapy was correcting a deficient diet, a few milligrams a day would be enough, but the dosages required to treat the problems I mentioned are fantastically large—anywhere from 20 to 500 times the RDA. We can't possibly get these amounts from food alone, even from the most well-balanced, nutrient-rich diet imaginable. So it's not that we are getting less B_6 than before; apparently, many of us simply need a lot more B_6 than our grandparents did.

There are two possible ways in which our need for vitamin B_6 might have increased. One could be through a genetic mutation, though such major evolutionary changes usually require thousands or millions of years to be completed. The other possibility is that changes in our environment (particularly environmental pollution and food processing) have affected the way our bodies handle this vitamin. There is reason to believe that these environmental changes are indeed causing trouble.

Antimetabolites Are the Culprits

Any substance that interferes with the metabolism or functioning of a nutrient is called an antimetabolite, or an antagonist. An antimetabolite of vitamin B₆ might act in any one of several different ways: It might prevent B₆ from being absorbed, inhibit its passage from the blood to the cells, cause its breakdown or rapid excretion, or inhibit its usual biochemical functions. If these antimetabolites do exist, we would need to increase our B₆ intake to counteract their effects.

There is evidence that vitamin B₆ antagonists have become an integral part of modern living and that we have been exposed to increasing amounts during the past 30 years. Chemicals that interfere with vitamin B₆ are used extensively in industry as antitarnish agents, as plating materials and in metal manufacturing. Modern food processing generates vitamin B₆ antagonists in our food. At least one widely used food coloring, several herbicides and plant-growth regulators that contaminate our food are also suspected B₆ antimetabolites. Even some prescription medications cause vitamin B₆ deficiency. Because we are being bombarded with antimetabolites from all directions, it's no wonder that more and more of us need greater and greater amounts of B₆. The long-term consequences of this environmental and dietary pollution are unknown, although certainly not encouraging.

The list of known or suspected vitamin B₆ antimetabolites represents just the tip of the iceberg. Many more of the thousands of chemicals in our environment will probably be found to interfere with B₆ or some other essential nutrient. With the proliferation of antimetabolites may come new diseases and ever-increasing needs for particular vitamins or minerals.

Here are the substances known or suspected to interfere with our bodies' metabolism of vitamin B₆.

Hydrazines and Hydrazides

A widely used group of chemicals called hydrazines and hydrazides appears to be a major threat to our vitamin B₆ metabolism. Hydrazines and hydrazides contain a pair of nitrogen molecules bound to each other and are structurally similar to pyridoxine (vitamin B_6). Biochemists will tell you that a chemical whose structure resembles a particular vitamin will often interfere with the function of that vitamin.

A group of Italian scientists studied how various chemicals affect vitamin B_6 metabolism. They found that all compounds with a free hydrazine group strongly inhibited vitamin B_6–dependent enzymes.[7,8] Bela Toth, Ph.D., of the University of Nebraska Medical Center, has also studied the relationship between hydrazines and vitamin B_6.[9] Various hydrazine compounds injected in mice caused convulsions and death; when the animals were also given pyridoxine, however, it completely prevented the toxic effects of four out of five hydrazines. Toxicity of the fifth compound was also partly prevented by B_6. Dr. Toth's work suggested that the adverse effects of various hydrazines are due at least partly to interference with vitamin B_6 metabolism.

A series of synthetic hydrazide compounds has also been studied by Canadian biochemists. Every chemical they tested reduced the activity of vitamin B_6–dependent enzymes.

The consequences of interfering with vitamin B_6–dependent enzymes can be appreciated only if we understand the crucial role that enzymes play in bodily functions. These versatile protein molecules catalyze thousands of different biochemical reactions. Without enzymes, many of the body's normal functions would cease. Properly functioning enzymes are necessary for good health and for life itself. Most enzymes, however, cannot perform alone—they must first be activated by another compound (usually a vitamin), called a coenzyme. As long as the coenzyme does its job, the enzyme will work properly. If there is an inadequate supply of coenzyme (that is, a vitamin deficiency), or if the coenzyme is somehow prevented from activating its counterpart enzyme, important biochemical reactions will break down, and we will become ill or die.

Hydrazines and hydrazides probably interfere with the function of enzymes that depend on vitamin B_6 by binding onto enzymes where B_6 would normally bind. With its "activating site" already occupied, B_6 is unable to activate its enzyme.

Vitamin B_6 is the coenzyme for more than 50 enzymes, so interference with B_6-dependent enzymes could lead to any number of metabolic abnormalities. It's no wonder that the epidemic of B_6 deficiency has surfaced in so many different guises.

Not all hydrazines and hydrazides in our environment have yet been tested for their effect on B_6 metabolism, but since so many of these chemicals are known antimetabolites, the others should be considered suspected offenders until proved otherwise.

Hydrazine

This chemical is frequently used as rocket fuel and in military aircraft like the F-16. Traces of hydrazine also appear in cigarette smoke. Hydrazine's greatest hazard is that it may cause cancer, but it's chemical structure strongly suggests that it's also a vitamin B_6 antagonist. Hydrazine injections produce epileptic seizures in animals that can be treated effectively with pyridoxine.[10] Because B_6 deficiency also causes seizures, hydrazine probably triggers seizures by interfering with vitamin B_6 metabolism. Our exposure to hydrazines and hydrazides is far less than the amount needed to induce convulsions in animals, but these chemicals could lead to more subtle problems with vitamin B_6 metabolism, even if they do not cause outright epilepsy.

Vitamin B_6 appears to be an antidote to human hydrazine poisoning. James K. Kirklin, M.D., and associates treated a 36-year-old man who had lapsed into a coma after being exposed to hydrazine in an industrial explosion. After receiving an injection of pyridoxine (25 milligrams per kilogram of body weight), the man improved rapidly.[10]

Some people—particularly those who live near military bases or launching pads—are exposed to hydrazines from air polluted with rocket or jet fuel. Hydrazine is relatively stable in air; traces persist for days or even weeks after it's released from the exhaust of a rocket or jet.[11]

Another major source of hydrazine exposure is tobacco and tobacco smoke,[12] since small amounts are found naturally in tobacco plants. Hydrazine also contaminates maleic hydrazide, a widely used sprouting inhibitor sprayed on tobacco plants. This means that cigarette smoking or tobacco chewing may increase our need for B_6. In a recent study, researchers compared the amounts of vitamin B_6 in the bodies of smoking and nonsmoking pregnant women.[13] Even though all the women consumed similar amounts of B_6, smokers had lower levels of the vitamin in their blood than nonsmokers. Forty-nine percent of the smokers, but only 23 percent of the nonsmokers, were deficient in B_6. The infants of smoking mothers in this study weighed 300 to 500 grams less than the infants of nonsmokers. The study also showed that if the smokers took an additional 15 milligrams of B_6 every day, they were less likely to give birth to an underweight baby. While there may be other factors in tobacco smoke that interfere with vitamin B_6, hydrazine and maleic hydrazide almost certainly contribute.

Isoniazid

Isoniazid (also known as isonicotinic acid hydrazide, or INH) is a drug used to prevent and treat tuberculosis. Although active tuberculosis has become much less common in the United States, prescriptions for isoniazid are by no means rare. Many people have been exposed to tuberculosis, even though they don't actually show symptoms. Depending on age and medical history, doctors advise some exposed people to take INH daily for a year or more to prevent a full-blown outbreak of the disease. Patients treated with isoniazid can develop vitamin B_6 deficiency[14] that is so severe in some cases that it produces an irreversible neuritis (inflammation of the nerves).[15] The neuritis is usually preventable if large amounts of B_6 are given along with the isoniazid therapy.

Isoniazid overdose can produce seizures, acidosis and even coma, but Maurice L. Sievers, M.D., who has treated more than 150 patients for isoniazid overdose, says intravenous pyridoxine is an effective antidote.[16]

Hydralazine

Hydralazine (a hydrazine compound) is a prescription medication used to treat high blood pressure or to dilate the blood vessels of heart patients. This drug is also a known B_6 antagonist,[17] and, like INH, it has caused some cases of peripheral neuritis.[18] Many patients who take hydralazine have heart disease. Since vitamin B_6 deficiency itself appears to contribute to heart disease, hydralazine could eventually aggravate a heart condition. Unless there is good reason to the contrary, anybody taking hydralazine should, with the approval of a physician, take a vitamin B_6 supplement.

Phenelzine

Phenelzine (phenylethylhydrazine) is an antidepressant. This hydrazine compound, another known B_6 antagonist,[19] has caused a number of cases of severe edema (swelling) in elderly patients.[20] The edema could have been due to vitamin B₆ deficiency, since swelling is one of the symptoms frequently associated with low levels of B₆. Depressed people can ill afford to develop B₆ deficiency as a side effect of their treatment. Indeed, as we shall see in chapter 4, lack of this vitamin actually *causes* some cases of depression. Fortunately, because of other potential dangers of phenelzine, the drug is not used very often.

Maleic Hydrazide

This compound is used as a plant-growth inhibitor and herbicide. It's sprayed primarily on tobacco but is also used on other crops, such as potatoes and onions.[19] The concentration of maleic hydrazide in potatoes ranged in one study from 5.3 to 8.3 parts per million.[21] This chemical becomes concentrated to a much greater degree when potatoes are made into potato chips. Currently, United States regulations allow up to 160 parts per million of maleic hydrazide in potato chips.[19] At that concentration, a mere 2 ounces of potato chips would provide more than 8 milligrams of unwanted maleic hydrazide. It's impossible to tell just how dangerous that level of exposure is. Although we don't know for sure whether maleic hydrazide is a vitamin B₆ antagonist, we do know that it's similar in structure to other hydrazides that interfere with B₆. Because exposure to this chemical is so great (some of us ingest more maleic hydrazide each day than vitamin B₆), studies on its relationship to B₆ are urgently needed.

Succinic Acid 2, 2-Dimethylhydrazide

This chemical is used in the United States and Canada. Peaches, nectarines, tomatoes, brussels sprouts, cherries, grapes and apples are sprayed with this compound, since food scientists have found that they can lower production costs by shortening the ripening period for fruits. This chemical enables farmers to harvest a tree once and only once with a mechanical device.[22] Unfortunately, residues of this ripening agent persist in the fruit.

Tartrazine

Also known as FD&C Yellow No. 5, tartrazine is a coloring agent added to foods and prescription medications since 1916. This widely used dye is found in hundreds of different foods and in more than 300 drugs and vitamin preparations.[23] As of 1983, nearly 1.5 million pounds of tartrazine were being used annually. Most people ingest this dye every day, and some diets contain up to 7.5 milligrams a day[24] (the average daily intake of B_6 is less than 2 milligrams). Tartrazine itself is not a hydrazine, but animal studies have shown that at least 30 percent of ingested tartrazine is converted by the body to 4-sulphophenylhydrazine, a hydrazine compound.[25] We cannot rule out the possibility that other food dyes with similar chemical structures may also be converted to hydrazine compounds inside the body. Modern processed foods and prescription drugs containing FD&C Yellow No. 5 are yet another source of vitamin B_6 antagonists.

Other Vitamin B$_6$ Antagonists

Although hydrazines and hydrazides are widespread and potent inhibitors of vitamin B_6, they are not the only substances threatening our bodies' use of B_6. Many nonhydrazine compounds—including various prescription medications, industrial chemicals and by-products of food processing—have been introduced into our environment during modern times. It's likely that they, too, are contributing to the epidemic of vitamin B_6 dependency. Here are a few cases in point.

Medications

Birth control pills,[26] penicillamine (used for the treatment of rheumatoid arthritis and lead poisoning)[27] and cycloserine (used to treat tuberculosis)[28] can contribute to B_6 deficiency.

The Pill, which is taken by an estimated 10 million American women, seems to be a common cause of vitamin B_6 deficiency, which can lead to depression or abnormal glucose tolerance. We shall also see how inadequate supplies of this vitamin can contribute to pregnancy complications, such as nausea and vomiting, toxemia or diabetes. Low levels of B_6 in pregnant mothers can also interfere with the growth and health of newborns.

Studies at the Department of Foods and Nutrition at Purdue University showed that women who had used the Pill before becoming pregnant had lower B_6 levels in their own blood and in the blood of their fetuses than did women who had not taken the Pill.[29] Nutritionally aware doctors advise all women using oral contraceptives to supplement their B_6 intake by at least 10 or 20 milligrams a day.

Polychlorinated Biphenyls

Polychlorinated biphenyls (PCB's) are a group of synthetic organic compounds used in industry. They have been used in the electrical industry to produce capacitors and transformers, and have been employed in heat-exchange systems, hydraulic fluids and lubricants. In the past, many consumer products also contained PCB's.

These chemicals are highly toxic. They have caused defects in the immune system, digestive disturbances, skin lesions, impotence, birth defects and liver disorders.[30-33] Because they were also found to cause cancer, in 1976 the government banned further production of PCB's. Unfortunately, PCB's that were already in use were not banned, and they remain in the environment in disturbingly large amounts. PCB's can now be found in the bodies of over 99 percent of all Americans and in 100 percent of Canadians.[32]

Industrial wastes in our waters have contaminated the food chain with PCB's. Fish often contain PCB's and are now considered to be our primary source of exposure, although other foods at the top of the food chain (such as meat, poultry, eggs and milk) may also be important sources. Because these chemicals are highly soluble in fat, they tend to collect in fatty tissues and become concentrated at the top of the food chain. In a 1975 survey, PCB's were detected in 69 percent of breast milk samples analyzed, and 30 percent of the samples had concentrations greater than 0.5 parts per million.[30] In Michigan, where environmental PCB contamination has been a serious problem, high PCB levels in fish required that controls be put on commercial fishing. In a 1977–78 survey of breast milk from more than 1,000 nursing mothers in Michigan, 100 percent was contaminated with PCB's. In some women the concentration was as high as 5 parts per million.[30]

In addition to their other toxic effects, PCB's may also cause problems with vitamin B_6 metabolism. Japanese scientists fed rats PCB's for four weeks at concentrations ranging from 10 to 100 milligrams per kilogram of body weight per day. They found that PCB's lowered the amount of pyridoxal phosphate (the biologically active form of B_6) in the liver.[33] Although the amount of PCB's needed to reduce B_6 levels in rats is higher than the amounts to which humans are normally exposed,

PCB's effects, when added to those of other B_6 antagonists, may turn out to be more significant than we realize.

By-products of Food Processing

The typical American diet has lost perhaps 50 percent or more of its vitamin B_6 content due to refining of sugar and whole grains, canning of vegetables, overheating of meats and other processing techniques. Many of us don't even consume the RDA for vitamin B_6. Even if we did, there would still be other problems with our diet.

Overheated vegetable oil seems to be a major culprit in depleting B_6. In the nineteenth century, nearly everyone cooked and baked with butter or lard. It wasn't until around 1925 that vegetable oil became a significant source of calories in our diet. As the medical community became convinced that polyunsaturated fats could protect our hearts, corn oil, safflower oil and other vegetable oils were ingrained in our minds as the "healthy fats." The chapter on heart disease points out that these vegetable oils may not be the answer to preventing heart disease. Vegetable oils that have been used for frying are the least healthful. It seems that when these oils are heated excessively, toxic by-products are produced that interfere with vitamin B_6 metabolism.

Because of their chemical structure, the unsaturated fats in vegetable oils are easily oxidized. At high temperatures, oxidation proceeds much more rapidly than usual. Vegetable oil heated in the presence of oxygen (the air in a typical room contains about 20 percent oxygen) undergoes major chemical changes, possibly producing peroxides and other toxins. In 1954 Lloyd A. Witting and co-workers at the University of Illinois fed rats corn oil that had been used to fry potato chips.[34] This frying oil made up 10 percent of the total diet, the amount many of us normally consume. Witting found that rats fed the frying oil grew more slowly than rats given a similar amount of fresh corn oil. However, when the rats fed on frying oil also consumed vitamin B_6 (10 milligrams per kilogram of diet), they grew faster. The vitamin did not, on the other hand, improve the growth of rats given fresh oil. Something in the heated corn oil was stunting the rats' growth.

Witting's findings may have profound implications for human health. It's true that heated vegetable oils are only one more item on the seemingly endless list of B_6 antagonists, but because of the massive amounts we consume, these oils must be put near the top of the list of offending agents. In 1953 more than 172 million pounds of oil were heated to between 340° and 400°F to produce potato chips alone. When we add to this the millions of pounds of oil used for making french fries, fried chicken and the countless other fried and baked goods that find their way into our homes, restaurants and fast-food stores, our total consumption becomes alarmingly high. Some commercial frying oil is used over and over again. Hour after hour, it sits in the open air at exceedingly high temperatures, becoming more and more toxic as the day wears on. Some restaurants never throw away old oil; they merely add a fresh supply as the level in the fryer falls. It is hard to imagine a more likely way to ruin your health than to eat the peroxides this produces. People who overdo it on fried foods are probably getting 10 percent or more of their calories from dangerous oils, and their diet alone may be enough to cause problems with B_6 metabolism. For others, smaller quantities provide an additional burden to a delicate biochemistry already threatened by other antimetabolites.

It's not certain how heated oil interferes with vitamin B_6. We do know that various types of processed fats can make us deficient in essential fatty acids (EFA's), and that vitamin B_6 metabolism is closely tied to EFA's. We also know that extra B_6 will reduce the damage caused by a diet low in EFA's; conversely, EFA supplements will prevent some of the damage caused by a B_6-deficient diet. Whatever the mechanism, prudence dictates that we avoid fried vegetable oil.

From our discussion so far, potato chips emerge as a highly suspect food. Not only have they been drenched in oil, but they may contain up to 160 parts per million of maleic hydrazide. Although no one has yet made a careful study, it wouldn't be surprising to find that potato chip "abusers" suffer more frequently than others from some of the B_6-responsive disorders discussed in this book.

There are at least two other components of processed food that interfere with vitamin B_6 metabolism. One of these is caramel color, a food additive produced by heating sugars. Caramel color inhibits pyridoxal kinase, an enzyme that converts B_6 into its biologically active form (pyridoxal phosphate). In test tube studies, this food additive somehow prevented pyridoxine (another form of B_6) from traveling into brain tissue.[35]

The other component of processed food that seems to affect vitamin B_6 is pyridoxyl-lysine.[36] This compound is produced during heat processing and storage of various foods. Pyridoxyl-lysine (abbreviated PL) is made up of a vitamin B_6 molecule and a lysine molecule. The latter is one of the essential amino acids present in most protein-containing foods. Harsh processing and storage can link these two molecules together. Scientists have found that high doses of PL could satisfy the nutritional requirement for vitamin B_6. Low doses, on the other hand, can create the need for more B_6. Exactly why different amounts of PL had different effects is not clear. However, human beings are more likely to be exposed to small rather than large amounts of this molecule, so it's possible that processed food interferes with B_6 in yet another way.

Naturally Occurring Vitamin B_6 Antagonists

Several vitamin B_6 antagonists are known to occur naturally in food. A hydrazine compound named linatine has been identified in linseed (flaxseed) meal.[37] When animals eat linseed meal as a main dietary staple, the resulting B_6 deficiency can retard their growth. Adding extra vitamin B_6 to the animals' diet can prevent stunted growth.

A suspected B_6 antagonist called agaritine has been found in the commonly eaten mushroom *Agaricus bisporus* (known as button mushrooms).[19] Agaritine is a hydrazine, so it must be considered an antimetabolite until proved otherwise. These mushrooms contain up to 400 parts per million of agaritine. At this concentration, one could easily obtain several milligrams of agaritine in a normal serving. Americans consumed approximately 350 million pounds of this mushroom in 1975.

A third compound that interferes with B_6 is called L-canaline.[38] While this chemical doesn't normally appear in food, it can be manufactured from L-canavanine, a compound present in alfalfa seeds and sprouts. The safety of alfalfa sprouts, long thought of as a prime example of health food, must therefore be reconsidered and studied more fully. Already there is evidence that feeding enormously large amounts of dried alfalfa sprouts to monkeys produces an illness similar to the severe autoimmune disease lupus erythematosus.[39]

Protecting Ourselves, Our Environment

An epidemic of vitamin B_6 deficiency has emerged in the past several decades, probably triggered by food processing, environmental pollution and certain prescription medications. The wide range of seemingly unrelated disorders known to improve with B$_6$ therapy indicates how much our environment interferes with vitamin B$_6$ metabolism.

To the extent that toxins in our environment are making us ill, perhaps vitamin therapy can reduce the damage. Unless we control the problems of chemical pollution and adulteration of our food, we will eventually see diseases that even the best nutritional program can't cure. Perhaps the story of vitamin B$_6$ will make us more aware of the extent to which the environment can affect our bodies' biochemistry.

Why the RDA Is Irrelevant

The RDA for B$_6$ is 2 milligrams a day for the average adult female, 2.2 milligrams a day for the average adult male, and 2.6 and 2.5 milligrams for pregnant and lactating women, respectively (slightly larger amounts are recommended with high-protein diets). However, the Committee on Dietary Allowances of the National Research Council, the group that developed the RDA's, admits that these allowances apply only to healthy people. Premature babies and people with infections, inherited metabolic disorders or chronic diseases, as well as anyone taking medication[40] may need more B$_6$ than the RDA. When you consider how widespread chronic fatigue, depression, hyperactivity, allergies, arthritis, cancer, cardiovascular disease and diabetes are, it becomes apparent that the RDA's are not relevant for the majority of Americans. Indeed, as Professor Roger Williams has pointed out,[41] some people may be ill precisely *because* they have an unusually large nutritional need that isn't being met.

Because we consume nutrient-depleted food and are exposed to antimetabolites, it's logical to suppose that we could use more B$_6$ than we are getting. But how could some of us need 25 or even 100 times the RDA? These are far greater amounts than one could ever obtain from food alone.

The discovery of the so-called vitamin B$_6$ dependency syndromes was the first indication that humans could inherit an unusually large need for B$_6$. At least five metabolic abnormalities that respond to vitamin B$_6$ supplements have been reported:[42] B$_6$-dependent convulsions, B$_6$-responsive anemia, cystathioninuria, xanthurenic aciduria and homocystinuria. In each of these disorders, several of which may be characterized by mental retardation, large amounts of B$_6$ are needed to correct a metabolic abnormality. It's possible that the vitamin B$_6$ dependency syndromes are only the tip of the iceberg. How many of us are ill because of a mild vitamin B_6 dependency that has been brought to the surface by antimetabolite exposure?

Vitamin B_6 requirements could increase as a result of any number of metabolic defects. Absorption of the vitamin may be poor, or there may be a problem transporting it from the blood into the brain or other tissues. Some people may have trouble converting pyridoxine into its active form, pyridoxal phosphate. Others may have an abnormal enzyme that can't bind to B_6 unless larger amounts of the vitamin are present. Still others may have enzymes that are unusually susceptible to destruction unless they are "protected" by large quantities of B_6. As we learn more about nutrition and biochemistry, we will probably become more aware of how subtle biochemical changes can affect our vitamin needs. Perhaps some of us have inherited an unusual sensitivity to B_6 antimetabolites. This may explain why some people can thrive in a toxic environment that makes other people vulnerable to illness.

Inhibition and Induction

Most antimetabolites act by blocking the site on an enzyme where the coenzyme (vitamin) usually binds. This interference by the antimetabolite prevents activation of the enzyme. Depending on how an antimetabolite combines with the enzyme, its inhibiting effect may be called either *competitive* or *noncompetitive*. Competitive inhibition can be reversed by flooding the system with more of the vitamin. A large amount of B_6 will compete more effectively than a small amount for binding sites on the enzyme. In a sense, the extra B_6 drives the antagonist away, activating the enzyme again. Many B_6 antimetabolites are extremely potent; that is, they are much better competitors for the enzyme than are the vitamins. A hydrazine compound might, for example, bind 100 times more tightly than vitamin B_6. Consequently, it would take many B_6 molecules to counteract the effect of a single antimetabolite molecule. Genetic factors may also be involved. For example, some people may have inherited an enzyme that is unusually susceptible to the damaging effect of an antimetabolite.

Noncompetitive inhibitors can't simply be driven away. Once an enzyme comes in contact with a noncompetitive inhibitor, that enzyme is out of action for good. If enough vitamin B_6 is present, however, it can counteract a noncompetitive inhibitor by stimulating the body to manufacture more enzyme molecules. This process is called *enzyme induction*. When large amounts of B_6 are present, the machinery that produces B_6-dependent enzymes somehow speeds up (or perhaps the rate of destruction slows down).

How can you determine what the best dose of B_6 is for you? Unfortunately, there is no reliable way to tell for sure. Several lab tests are used, especially by researchers, to detect vitamin B_6 deficiency or dependency, but laboratory tests alone can't always give an accurate picture of our B_6 requirements.

One frequently used biochemical test for B_6 deficiency is the tryptophan load test. When the body is low in B_6, tryptophan is converted to certain abnormal by-products, including xanthurenic acid. Excretion of these by-products after ingestion of tryptophan is taken as evidence of vitamin B_6 deficiency.[43] The results of this test must be interpreted carefully, since a normal tryptophan load test does not guarantee that B_6 levels are optimal. For instance, there are many B_6-dependent enzymes that have nothing to do with tryptophan metabolism. A tryptophan load test would fail to detect B_6 deficiencies that arise when one of these enzymes is genetically weak or is attacked by an antimetabolite. Likewise, an abnormal test doesn't prove B_6 deficiency. Some scientists have argued, for example, that the increased excretion of xanthurenic acid in women who take birth control pills is not necessarily caused by lack of B_6. Despite its limitations, the tryptophan load test can provide useful information if it's interpreted carefully.

Another test of B_6 deficiency measures the activity of a B_6-dependent enzyme in red blood cells. The activity of this enzyme (erythrocyte glutamic oxalacetic transaminase, abbreviated EGOT) is measured in the test tube before and after vitamin B_6 is added.[43,44] In normal people with no B_6 deficiency, most of the EGOT is already activated, and adding more B_6 to the test tube will not increase the EGOT activity. On the other hand, if someone is deficient in B_6, fewer EGOT enzymes would be activated, and adding B_6 to the test tube would increase the enzyme's activity. According to some scientists, vitamin B_6 deficiency exists when adding the vitamin to the test tube increases EGOT activity more than 25 percent. Since this test measures only 1 of the more than 50 B_6-dependent enzymes, it may fail to detect some cases of B_6 dependency.

Other tests used to assess B_6 status include measuring blood levels of pyridoxal phosphate or urinary excretion of 4-pyridoxic acid (a breakdown product of vitamin B_6). While these tests are sensitive enough to detect an outright B_6 deficiency, they can't determine whether someone has an unusually large need for the vitamin. So although laboratory tests may provide some information, there is no foolproof way of determining how much B$_6$ you need.

At present, most nutrition-oriented doctors prescribe vitamin B$_6$ on the basis of clinical experience and common sense. If you are basically healthy, it would probably be a good idea to supplement your diet with 10 or 20 milligrams of this vitamin as part of an overall nutritional program. Remember, nutrients work better when supplied as a team than when taken individually. If you have an illness that might be related to vitamin B$_6$, larger doses may be necessary. Although there seems to be little danger in taking up to 50 milligrams of this vitamin a day, you should consult with your doctor before using B$_6$ as therapy.

Part II
Women's Special Needs

Chapter

The Premenstrual 2
Syndrome

Mrs. M. a 32-year-old mother of two, came to my office a little more than a year ago for a general checkup. She had been basically healthy since childhood and did not have any particular medical problems. In fact, she said she usually felt fine. Like so many other women, however, there was one group of symptoms that she had not thought to mention, even though they had plagued her for nearly 20 years. Evidently, Mrs. M. did not consider the bloated abdomen and the headaches she suffered for two days before each menstrual period to be true "symptoms." Nor did she feel that the swelling in her hands and breasts or the severe anxiety she also developed around this time were worth mentioning. Having suffered with these problems for so long, she had simply resigned herself to the fact that she was going to feel rotten for two days out of every month.

On one occasion Mrs. M. had mentioned her premenstrual symptoms to the gynecologist, who told her it was "just hormones." Her doctor had assured her that these symptoms were very common and that there was nothing to worry about.

It was only after I asked Mrs. M. specifically about symptoms related to her menstrual period that I learned about her monthly woes, which turned out to be rather severe. Two days before each menstrual period, Mrs. M. would develop gradually worsening tension and irritability. By the second day her nerves would be so frazzled that she would have difficulty coping with even the simplest daily chores. She would make mistakes at work, burst into tears for no reason and generally become unpleasant to be around. She would scream at her children and argue with her husband about matters of little importance. Mrs. M.'s premenstrual behavior had affected her marital relationship so much that her husband had several times threatened to leave her. The only reason he had put up with his wife during these times was that he knew she would be back to normal within a day or two.

Mrs. M. also complained of premenstrual headaches so severe that she would have to stay home from work and lie in bed all day. Her hands would get so puffy she couldn't even close them. As soon as her menstrual period began, however, all of her symptoms would disappear with remarkable speed.

I had seen many women with symptoms similar to those that plagued Mrs. M. Most of these women had found considerable relief by taking large amounts of vitamin B_6, so I asked Mrs. M. to begin using 50 milligrams of B_6 twice daily and to return after three months. Although she could detect no change in symptoms during the first month, she noticed a dramatic improvement by the second menstrual period—no more mood swings, arguments, crying spells or errors at work. Her headaches, though still present, were only mild and quite tolerable. The bloating in her abdomen, breasts and hands was also considerably reduced. Mrs. M. remarked that her relationship with her husband had improved, too. For the first time that she could remember, she did not look to the end of each cycle with dread. After experimenting with the dosage for six months, Mrs. M. learned that 50 milligrams of vitamin B_6 once daily was sufficient to control her premenstrual symptoms. If she discontinued the vitamin altogether, however, her problems would return in full force the following month.

The Neglected Syndrome

Mrs. M.'s case is typical of the premenstrual syndrome (PMS), a symptom complex that appears to affect a large percentage of women. Although this common and often troublesome syndrome is probably as old as the human race, and although it had been described in the medical literature more than 50 years ago, it has until recently been largely ignored by the medical profession. There are several reasons for the relative lack of interest in PMS. One is that many doctors did not believe the syndrome really existed. They assumed that symptoms that could not be explained scientifically were not real. Doctors knew that many women have no problems at all with their menstrual periods. Those who complained were therefore passed off as neurotic, in need of psychiatric, rather than medical, therapy.

Another reason for the lack of interest is that doctors who did accept PMS's existence considered it a natural part of the human reproductive cycle, a result of normal monthly hormonal fluctuations. Many physicians figured that some women were simply destined to feel bad at certain times of the month, and there was nothing to be done about it. After all, hadn't women managed with these symptoms since the beginning of time? Why shouldn't modern women also make it through their menstrual cycle? It was even suggested as recently as 1974 that PMS was programmed by evolutionary forces to discourage the male, through hostile behavior, from wasting his sexual energies at a time when conception would not be possible. Most doctors accepted the more likely explanation that PMS is caused by hormonal imbalances; however, few of them assigned much importance to their patients' complaints.

Doctors have recently received a great deal of criticism about their attitudes toward women's health care. They have been accused, apparently with some justification, of failing to take seriously women's legitimate medical needs. For example, according to one recent study published in the *Journal of the American Medical Association*,[1] doctors were more likely to perform diagnostic tests if a man had certain complaints than if a woman had the same symptoms. All too often women's health problems have been brushed off either as insignificant, or as "all in the head."

The failure of doctors to provide adequate treatment for PMS is perhaps a prime example of the gripes that some women have had about modern medicine. Had there been more interest in the subject, perhaps researchers would have discovered long ago that vitamin B_6 supplements usually relieve many of the symptoms of PMS. Or perhaps they would have heard the lone voice of Katherina Dalton, M.D., the British physician who has been advocating for more than two decades the use of the natural hormone progesterone for PMS.

In the past several years, attitudes about PMS have begun to change, partly because physicians' attitudes toward women's health care have evolved. In addition, women themselves have become more assertive in the face of patronizing attitudes toward their problems. Then, too, new research has clearly shown that safe and effective treatments are available for PMS. For all these reasons, this long-neglected disorder is now the focus of increasing attention among both doctors and the public.

Most doctors now agree that PMS does exist and is a physical, rather than psychological, disorder. In a comprehensive review of the subject, S. S. C. Yen, M.D., of the Department of Reproductive Medicine, School of Medicine, University of California at San Diego, and Robert L. Reid, M.D., called PMS "a major clinical entity affecting a large segment of the female population."[2] Just how common this syndrome is has been a subject of debate. Questionnaires designed to determine the incidence of PMS may be somewhat misleading, because women with symptoms may be more likely to fill out and return the questionnaires than those who feel well. In addition, there may indeed be a psychological component to PMS, which would make interpretation of physical symptoms more difficult. For example, in one study, women reported more physical complaints when they were misled into believing they were in their premenstrual phase.[2] Despite these difficulties with arriving at a precise estimate, the consensus among gynecologists is that between 70 and 90 percent of females of childbearing age have recurrent premenstrual symptoms. The physical or emotional symptoms of an estimated 20 to 40 percent of these women are severe.

PMS symptoms usually begin several days to one week before menstruation, although some women experience difficulties as much as two weeks or more before their period. The symptoms often become more severe as the period approaches and then stop abruptly as soon as the menstrual flow starts. If the menstrual period is delayed for some reason, symptoms will continue and may even get worse. Common complaints include emotional tension and depression, headaches, weight gain and fluid retention, swollen breasts, bloated abdomen, nausea, constipation and eruptions of acne on the face or shoulders. Some women feel clumsy and accident-prone. Others report increased appetite and an intense craving for sweet or salty foods. In some women these symptoms are only mild, but in others they are so devastating that normal activity becomes impossible for several days.

Just how much our attitudes about this once neglected syndrome have changed is illustrated by the results of two recent court cases in Great Britain. In both cases PMS was successfully used as a legal defense, and a charge of murder was reduced to manslaughter. In each case the women were judged to have "diminished responsibility" during the premenstrual phase of their cycles.[3] Clearly, PMS has finally come out of the closet and is now recognized as a legitimate medical condition with potentially serious consequences.

A Search for Causes to Find Cures

As with other medical illnesses, scientists have attempted to discover the cause of PMS in order to develop effective treatments. At this point, although there are several different theories, no one has yet proved what is at the root of this common syndrome.

Some doctors believe that the symptoms of PMS are due to edema (fluid buildup). The edema is, in turn, caused by hormonal imbalance. Excess fluid in the intestines, for example, might easily produce a bloated feeling and nausea, just as fluid in the breasts would cause a sensation of swelling and tenderness. The headaches and psychological changes might also conceivably be related to edema in the brain tissue. If the edema theory is correct, then diuretics would provide relief from most or all of the symptoms of PMS. In fact, many physicians do prescribe these drugs for this purpose.

Because diuretics have the potential for causing harm by depleting the body of essential minerals, it is important that we evaluate carefully the evidence on which diuretic treatment is based. Although the fluid-retention concept seems reasonable on the surface, there is evidence that contradicts it. For example, six patients with a history of premenstrual migraine headaches were given an injection of certain hormones known to cause fluid retention. None of these patients experienced a migraine attack as would have been expected if fluid buildup were the cause of these headaches. Furthermore, in patients who routinely suffered from migraines premenstrually, diuretics did not prevent the headaches from occurring.[2] There have been several reports that diuretics alleviated the symptoms of PMS, but these reports should be viewed cautiously. The improvement that occurred in these studies may have been due to a "placebo effect" rather than to the diuretics themselves. It has been shown many times that premenstrual symptoms frequently get better when women are given a placebo (a dummy pill with no active ingredients). Various experiments have demonstrated that anywhere from 15 to 88 percent of women treated with a placebo show some improvement. Because the symptoms of PMS can be influenced this way, a new treatment can be considered effective only if it is found to work better than a placebo. Doctors in Sweden conducted one such study,[4] comparing the effect of placebo tablets with that of chlorthalidone, a commonly used diuretic. Both treatments reduced the symptoms, but the placebo actually worked better than the diuretic.

It appears, then, that swelling is not the cause of PMS, but is just one of the many symptoms. For this reason it's unwise to use diuretics routinely during the premenstrual time. Although they may relieve uncomfortable swelling in some people, diuretics are apparently ineffective for the other symptoms and they may even make things worse. In addition, these drugs may produce nutritional deficiencies by increasing urinary losses of magnesium, potassium and other essential nutrients. Furthermore, if diuretics are used chronically, they may even lose their ability to relieve edema. In fact, diuretic abuse can actually *cause* edema.[5] Fortunately, diuretics aren't necessary to treat PMS because, as we shall see, vitamin B_6 therapy is a safe and effective method of relieving not only the edema, but many of the other symptoms of PMS.

Most researchers agree that hormonal imbalance is at the root of PMS, but exactly which hormones are involved is unclear. One theory holds that PMS is caused by excess estrogen, resulting either from overproduction by the ovaries or from inadequate breakdown of this hormone by the liver. An oversupply of estrogen, according to this theory, causes fluid retention. Estrogen accumulation in the brain is also suggested as the cause of the psychological changes in PMS. In addition, excess estrogen is known to cause changes in glucose tolerance,[6] which may be responsible for the sweets craving that some women experience before their period.

Other research points the finger at progesterone deficiency as the cause of PMS. Progesterone is a hormone produced by the ovaries that opposes the effect of estrogen. Thus, either too much estrogen or too little of its antagonist, progesterone, may be at the root of PMS. Still other studies suggest that an excess of prolactin, a hormone secreted by the pituitary gland, may be related to PMS. Exactly how these hormone imbalances lead to the many symptoms that occur premenstrually is not yet known.

Additional evidence suggests that a deficiency of a group of molecules known as brain amines may also be involved in PMS. Brain amines contain an amine molecule, chemically similar to ammonia. These amines serve a wide range of functions in the nervous system and other tissues. One of these molecules, called serotonin, is low in many people suffering from certain psychological disturbances. It is possible that a fall in serotonin levels during the premenstrual phase contributes to the emotional disturbances that are a part of PMS.[2] Another brain amine called dopamine affects the way the kidneys excrete fluid. A premenstrual drop in dopamine could possibly cause premenstrual edema.[2]

To summarize, many but not all studies have found that too much estrogen and prolactin, and too little progesterone, dopamine and serotonin are associated with PMS. No one really understands yet how all of these various molecules interact to produce PMS.

B₆: A Treatment That Works

At this point we do know enough to make an important observation: Vitamin B_6 has an effect on every one of the hormones and amines mentioned above. In each case B_6 produces a change that would be expected to relieve, rather than worsen, the symptoms of PMS. For instance, vitamin B_6 reduces the level of prolactin, which is thought to be too high in PMS.[7] Vitamin B_6 also reverses some of the adverse effects of estrogen medication, such as abnormal glucose tolerance[6] and psychological depression.[8] Since estrogen levels may be excessive in women with PMS, and since B_6 blocks some of the effects of estrogen overdose, this vitamin might help prevent premenstrual symptoms. In addition, B_6 may increase levels of progesterone,[9] dopamine[10] and serotonin,[11] all of which are believed to be too low in women with PMS. Because this vitamin interacts favorably with all these compounds, it seems vitamin B_6 would be an ideal treatment for women with PMS.

It's always tempting to draw conclusions and devise theories based on work done in animals or in test tubes. Sometimes these theories turn out to be correct, and sometimes they are way off base. If we didn't form new ideas by building on what we know, medicine would never progress. On the other hand, if we accepted as fact any theory that sounded reasonable, the market would be inundated with worthless and possibly dangerous remedies. Based on what we know so far about the causes of PMS, vitamin B_6 looks like the "magic bullet" that might possibly be the answer for this monthly suffering. The only way to find out for sure whether B_6 works is to compare its effectiveness to that of a placebo. Fortunately, vitamin B_6 has been tested in this way and found to be of great benefit. Thanks to the carefully done studies by Guy E. Abraham, M.D., and Joel T. Hargrove, M.D., of Rolling Hills, California, more and more doctors are beginning to prescribe B_6 and to report in medical journals[12] on its effectiveness. It's likely that vitamin B₆ therapy will soon find its way into the textbooks and become an accepted treatment for PMS.

Before discussing the important work of Drs. Abraham and Hargrove, the use of vitamin B₆ should be put into historical perspective. Students of nutrition must be reminded that many of the "new discoveries" in the field are actually not new at all. Thousands of reports attesting to the value of nutritional therapy lie buried in the back issues of medical journals, gathering dust in medical libraries around the country. Some of these old therapies have been "rediscovered," like that of B₆ for PMS, but most of them continue to be ignored. It's essential that we give appropriate credit to these earlier scientists, not only because they deserve it, but because doing so will remind us how much we can learn by looking into the medical archives.

The Early Discoveries

In early work with PMS, the entire vitamin B complex, which of course includes vitamin B₆, was used. Although the benefits of this treatment may have been due solely to B₆, some of the other B vitamins may also have contributed. In order to cover all the bases, most doctors who now treat PMS prescribe moderate doses of the B complex, in addition to relatively large amounts of B₆.

In 1944 Morton S. Biskind, M.D., a pioneer in nutritional therapy, discovered that the premenstrual symptoms of many of his patients improved strikingly after he treated them with B-complex vitamins.[13] Dr. Biskind had decided to try B vitamins in these women because of a theory he had developed during his research. When he fed rats a diet lacking in B vitamins, their livers lost the ability to inactivate estrogen at the normal rate. Dr. Biskind concluded from this work that B vitamins are needed by the liver to perform its usual task of inactivating this female hormone. If the same situation applied to humans, women deficient in B vitamins would have too much estrogen in their bodies, because their livers would not break it down fast enough. Nutritionally deficient women would therefore be expected to have symptoms associated with excess estrogen, such as heavy menstrual flow, irregular bleeding, cystic breasts and premenstrual tension.

In the early 1940's, before food manufacturers began adding vitamins to white bread, an observant physician could frequently find patients who had symptoms of classic B-vitamin deficiency. Dr. Biskind saw many such patients in his practice. Their usual complaints were weakness, fatigue, irritability or confusion. When he examined these patients, Dr. Biskind would often find a red, inflamed tongue or cracking at the corners of the mouth. Treatment with B vitamins would eliminate these symptoms and skin lesions, indicating that the symptoms had been caused by vitamin deficiency.

Once Biskind connected B vitamins to estrogen metabolism, he began asking every patient with B-vitamin deficiency whether she had certain symptoms that might be related to estrogen excess. Of 39 women questioned, 37 did have such symptoms, including one or more of the following: menorrhagia (heavy menstrual flow), metrorrhagia (bleeding between menstrual periods), painful breasts and premenstrual tension. After treatment with B vitamins, there was usually prompt and dramatic improvement, not only in the symptoms of B-vitamin deficiency, but also in the gynecological complaints. Improvement was not limited to those patients who had been grossly malnourished before treatment. Fifty-two other patients without obvious B-vitamin deficiencies were given B vitamins for one or more gynecological complaints. In these women, too, there was usually prompt relief.

Despite Dr. Biskind's report, the use of B vitamins for PMS did not become popular. Several years after Biskind published his work, another study questioned whether B vitamins are really involved in estrogen metabolism. Doctors at Hadassah University Hospital in Jerusalem studied 14 women with B-vitamin deficiency and found that their estrogen levels were normal. Furthermore, these malnourished women were able to remove estrogen from their system just as fast as women who had no nutritional deficiencies.[14] This research led scientists to reject the idea that B vitamins are related to estrogen metabolism, and Dr. Biskind's work with PMS was forgotten.

More recent work has shown that Dr. Biskind was probably right all along. There is now good evidence, both from the laboratory and the clinic, that vitamin B_6 is an effective remedy for PMS. In retrospect, one might argue that it was incorrect for doctors to reject B-vitamin therapy solely on the basis of the Hadassah study. In the first place, no one is really sure that estrogen excess is the main cause of PMS. If estrogen is involved, it may not be the only factor. Perhaps B vitamins relieve PMS in some way that has nothing to do with inactivating estrogen. As I mentioned earlier, there are a number of other ways in which the B complex, and especially vitamin B_6, might be related to

PMS. B₆ may lower prolactin or increase progesterone, serotonin or dopamine, all of which might be helpful for PMS.

There is a lesson to be learned from the fact that an effective remedy lay buried for 40 years before it was revived. Doctors should not be so quick to reject the clinical observations made by their peers merely because these observations don't fit current scientific theories. Dr. Biskind had made an important discovery: that a nontoxic vitamin is useful for a common problem. This observation should have been followed up immediately with controlled studies, regardless of whether his theories made scientific sense. History will most likely determine that Dr. Biskind's clinical observations were correct, even though his reason for using B vitamins may not have been entirely valid. How many other nutritional therapies have been allowed to die because doctors didn't understand how they could possibly work?

Newer Research Breakthroughs

In the early 1970's, many years after Dr. Biskind's work had been forgotten, new information appeared that clarified the relationship between estrogen and vitamin B₆. The level of vitamin B₆ in the bodies of women taking birth control pills and eating a B₆-deficient diet was measured, using the tryptophan load test.[15] Daily dosages as high as 20 milligrams of B₆ (ten times the Recommended Dietary Allowance [RDA] for adult women) were necessary to restore their B₆ levels to normal. Further studies showed that the B₆ deficiency was caused by the estrogen in these birth control pills as well as by the diet. It seems that estrogen supplements prompt the body to manufacture more of an enzyme needed to break down tryptophan. This enzyme, called tryptophan oxygenase, requires B₆ to function. When more of the enzyme is produced, it apparently pulls vitamin B₆ away from other places in the body, causing a deficiency at these other sites. Thus, B-vitamin deficiency doesn't cause estrogen excess, as Biskind postulated, but rather B₆ deficiency is *caused by* an oversupply of this hormone.

One of the possible consequences of estrogen-induced B₆ deficiency is depression, a side effect that occurs commonly in women taking the Pill. This adverse psychological change is presumably caused by a deficiency of serotonin, a molecule normally present in the brain, which appears to act as an antidepressant. Serotonin is synthesized from the amino acid tryptophan in a series of steps that will occur only if adequate

B_6 is present. A vitamin B_6 deficiency can result in inadequate production of serotonin, which then could result in depression.

In 1973 P. W. Adams, M.D., and co-workers[8] conducted a series of studies on 22 depressed women whose symptoms were judged to be due to the Pill. Out of the 22, 11 showed biochemical evidence of vitamin B_6 deficiency. When these 11 women were given 20 milligrams of B_6 twice daily for two months, their depression lifted. Treatment with a placebo, on the other hand, did not relieve the depression. Out of the original 22 women, 11 were not deficient in B_6. In this group, treatment with the vitamin did not help the depression. This study demonstrated that estrogen could cause depression in some women by producing a B_6 deficiency, and that the symptoms could be reversed by giving B_6 supplements.

The women in Dr. Adams's study did not have PMS, but their B_6 deficiency aggravated the symptoms of hormonal imbalance. Adams's data therefore brought up the possibility that the hormonal fluctuations that cause PMS may also produce their effect by causing vitamin B_6 deficiency.

To test this possibility, Drs. Abraham and Hargrove[12] recruited 25 women with moderate or severe PMS. Each woman was studied for a total of six menstrual cycles. During three of these cycles, they received each day a single sustained-release tablet containing 500 milligrams of pyridoxine hydrochloride (vitamin B_6). During the other three cycles, they were given an inert placebo that appeared identical to the B_6 tablets. Throughout the entire six-month study, each woman kept a daily symptom diary. A total of 19 symptoms were rated every day using a four-point scale. The daily symptom score was determined by adding all the scores for each of the 19 symptoms.

The study used the conventional double-blind method; that is, neither the women with PMS nor those administering the medications knew which tablets contained B_6 and which were placebos. The double-blind design was crucial, since if B_6 is to be accepted as an effective remedy, it must be proved superior to a placebo.

When the code was broken at the end of the six months and everyone discovered which tablets were the "active" ones, vitamin B_6 had performed far better than the placebo. Twenty-one of the 25 subjects had lower premenstrual symptom scores while taking the vitamin than while taking the placebo. In each of these 21 women, the difference between B_6 and placebo was statistically significant. That is, it was highly improbable that the improvements during B_6 therapy were due merely to random changes in the monthly symptoms.

The study done by Drs. Abraham and Hargrove should be acceptable even to the purest of scientists and to the most skeptical of physicians. Patients were carefully screened so that only those with well-defined PMS were included. The double-blind design eliminated the possibility that a placebo effect was involved. The results were evaluated statistically, so it could be stated with reasonable certainty that the improvements were not due to chance. Drs. Abraham and Hargrove have therefore demonstrated clearly and simply, using the rigid conventions of science, that vitamin B_6 supplements prevent premenstrual symptoms from occurring in a large percentage of women who normally suffer from moderate or severe PMS.

Drs. Abraham and Hargrove did not discuss exactly which symptoms improve the most on B_6 therapy. This question was addressed, however, in an earlier study by G. D. Kerr, M.D., a British gynecologist.[16] A group of 70 women with various premenstrual symptoms was treated with vitamin B_6 in dosages ranging from 40 to 100 milligrams a day. Of those who complained of depression, 60 percent were cured or markedly improved by B_6. The percentages of women whose other common symptoms were cured or markedly improved were: edema and bloatedness, 60 percent; irritability, 56 percent; lethargy, 52 percent; lack of coordination, 27 percent; and breast tenderness, 52 percent. Of those who suffered from premenstrual headaches, 81 percent found relief while on B_6 therapy. In a separate report, B. Leonard Snider, M.D., and David F. Dieteman, M.D., of Erie, Pennsylvania, gave 50 milligrams of B_6 daily to 106 girls who suffered from premenstrual acne flare-ups. Seventy-two percent of these girls noticed a lessening of premenstrual acne while on B_6.[17]

These figures provide a rough estimate of which symptoms are most likely to improve during vitamin B_6 therapy. Of course, patients in these studies were not given a placebo, so it's possible that some of the improvements were psychological. On the other hand, the B_6 dosages used (100 milligrams a day or less) were far less than the 500-milligram daily dose used by Drs. Abraham and Hargrove. Perhaps some of the women who failed to respond to the lower doses would have done better with more B_6.

The Question of Dosage

It may be hard to believe that such massive amounts of a vitamin would be necessary to correct PMS. After all, even the "low" dose of

100 milligrams a day is 50 times the RDA for vitamin B_6. In my experience, most women with a mild or moderate case of PMS can control their symptoms by taking 50 milligrams of B_6 a day. Some women do well with 20 milligrams. Nevertheless, an occasional patient will not obtain relief unless she consistently takes very large doses (but only under the guidance of a physician).

I recently consulted with R.P., a 27-year-old woman whose main problem was that she became extremely tense and irritable just before her menstrual period. For her, PMS was a great burden. She had an important job that required her to be pleasant and on her toes at all times. Unfortunately, for two days each month she felt "nasty and clumsy." At these times she became so hard to get along with that she would call in sick rather than come to work and risk injury to her professional reputation.

In addition to her premenstrual symptoms, R.P. also had frequent episodes of numbness, tingling, pain and weakness in the fingers of both hands. These symptoms often woke her up at night and bothered her frequently during the day. She noticed that only the thumb, the first two fingers, and half the ring finger on each hand caused problems. The other one and a half fingers felt normal. Although I didn't do nerve conduction studies to prove the diagnosis, the location of her symptoms strongly suggested that she was suffering from carpal tunnel syndrome, caused by compression of the median nerve as it travels past the wrist into the hand. The carpal tunnel syndrome (discussed in chapter 13) appears in many cases to be caused by vitamin B_6 deficiency.

R.P. was experiencing two common disorders, both of which usually respond to vitamin B_6 therapy. This patient had done a lot of reading about nutrition, and she was well aware of the importance of vitamin B_6. She had begun taking this vitamin about seven months previously. When her initial daily dosage of 100 milligrams didn't relieve her symptoms after a month, she increased the dose to 200 milligrams a day. (You should not take amounts this large without consulting your doctor.) When I first saw her she had been taking 200 milligrams of B_6 every day for six months without the slightest relief either in her premenstrual tension or the symptoms in her hands.

If 200 milligrams of vitamin B_6 was going to work, it would surely have done so in less than six months. B_6 usually relieves carpal tunnel syndrome within 12 weeks or less, and PMS usually responds even faster. Since it was obvious that 200 milligrams was not working, I asked R.P. to double the dose and return in two months. Within a month of taking 200 milligrams of B_6 twice daily she noticed considerable relief from both of her problems. She has remained free from symptoms over the past four months while continuing the larger dose of B_6.

It's not clear why R.P. needs so much B_6. Perhaps this is another example of vitamin B_6 dependency (see chapter 1) in which the body needs massive amounts of B_6 to overcome an inherited enzyme defect. Exactly how a genetic defect could produce the symptoms R.P. experienced is unclear. A wide range of symptoms can occur as a result of defects in enzymes that work together with vitamin B_6; however, in many of these cases, massive doses of B_6 have eliminated the symptoms. R.P. may also be especially sensitive to those environmental pollutants and processed foods that increase the need for B_6. Whatever the reason, this patient didn't feel well until she increased her B_6 dose to 400 milligrams a day.

How Safe Are Large Doses?

The issue of toxic dosages often arises in connection with vitamin therapy. Fortunately, vitamin B_6 appears to be quite safe in the dose range that is usually effective for PMS. So far, no severe side effects have been reported, even in patients taking as much as 800 milligrams a day, the amount sometimes prescribed for severe cases. We should not assume that B_6 is 100 percent safe at any dose level, however. Recent reports (see chapter 20) of nerve damage in seven people who took about 2,000 milligrams or more daily for more than a month should introduce a note of caution into vitamin B_6 therapy. Even though the vitamin was never proved to be the cause of the nerve damage, similar problems have been provoked in animals by feeding them massive amounts of B_6. No one should take more than 50 milligrams a day except under the guidance of a doctor familiar with B_6.

If side effects occur at doses under 100 milligrams a day, they are almost always mild and not dangerous. Some women find that they cannot take large amounts of B_6 because it gives them insomnia or makes them feel "wired" or "spaced-out." If the full dose is taken in the morning, the insomnia can sometimes be prevented. Also, some of these reactions to vitamin B_6 may be eliminated if a magnesium supplement is added to the diet.[18] Even though vitamin B_6 therapy seems safe, you should consult your doctor before going on a long-term supplement program. In addition, it's best to find the lowest dose that relieves your symptoms, rather than taking huge amounts of B_6 just for "insurance." Even though B_6 appears to be safe at present, vitamin therapy has not been around long enough for us to say for sure that large doses taken over a long time are entirely safe.

The Progesterone Connection

A brief word is in order concerning the relationship between vitamin B_6 and the natural hormone progesterone. Although it has not been proved by double-blind studies, most specialists in PMS are convinced that progesterone suppositories are extremely effective. Progesterone therapy is now being used for some patients in conjunction with vitamin B_6, diet modification, exercise and counseling.

Based on what we know about the chemistry of B_6, it seems that the effectiveness of this vitamin in PMS may be due, at least in part, to the relationship between B_6 and progesterone. According to a study[9] performed about 30 years ago, pregnant rats were unable to complete their pregnancies if they were fed a diet deficient in vitamin B_6. But when these B_6-deficient rats were also given injections of estrogen and progesterone, most of their pregnancies proceeded normally. Estrogen injections alone were not enough to save the pregnancies; progesterone was essential. This study demonstrated that vitamin B_6 deficiency reduces the production of or the effectiveness of progesterone. Perhaps in some cases of severe PMS a combination of progesterone and vitamin B_6 will be found to be more effective than either treatment alone.

The discovery that PMS can be relieved by vitamin B_6 has been an exciting one for nutrition-oriented health care practitioners everywhere. We are indeed fortunate to have a simple, safe, inexpensive and effective remedy for such a widespread problem. It may take a little more time before vitamin B_6 is used routinely by those doctors who are skeptical about nutritional therapy. At this time, however, more and more physicians are beginning to follow the lead of Drs. Biskind, Adams, Kerr and Abraham. Two review articles on PMS have appeared in medical publications in which the work of Biskind and Abraham was cited,[3,19] and both authors agreed that vitamin B_6 is useful in the treatment of PMS. It will not be long before the word gets around.

Chapter

Pregnancy 3

Most expectant mothers find that bringing a child into the world can be exciting, and the anticipation of creating a new life and a new member of the family can be joyous. Pregnancy is a complex biological function, though, and it exerts major stresses on the physiology of the mother. Her hormone levels fluctuate, and her nutritional requirements are increased by the demands of the growing fetus. Whether pregnancy proceeds normally or is attended by a host of complications depends on many different factors. Hundreds of scientific studies have shown that the mother's nutrition is key.

Malnutrition during pregnancy can impair fetal brain development, resulting in offspring of subnormal intelligence. Poor nutrition may also increase the risk of birth defects. An inadequate diet may adversely affect the mother's health as well.

All pregnant women need adequate amounts of protein, carbohydrates, fiber, fats, vitamins and minerals. No single nutrient is more important than any others. To assure a sufficient supply of nutrients during pregnancy, women should emphasize the use of whole foods, such as whole grains, beans, fresh fruits and vegetables, nuts and seeds, dairy products, eggs, fish, chicken and meat. Empty calories, found in sugar, refined flour, fatty and overprocessed foods, should be avoided. Since the additional need for iron during pregnancy cannot be met by diet alone, the Committee on Dietary Allowances of the Food and

Nutrition Board of the National Research Council has advised pregnant women to take a daily supplement containing 30 to 60 milligrams of iron.[1] Many obstetricians also prescribe multivitamin and multimineral supplements to increase their patients' daily intake of folic acid, calcium and other nutrients.

Do Expectant Mothers Need B_6?

The need for vitamin B_6 supplements during pregnancy is not widely recognized, despite considerable data showing its value. The Committee on Dietary Allowances recommends that pregnant women consume a mere 2.6 milligrams of B_6 a day. This slight increase over the usual Recommended Dietary Allowance (RDA) is based on the finding that women need to increase protein consumption by about 68 percent during pregnancy. The need for B_6 is directly related to the amount of protein in the diet—the more protein you eat, the more B_6 you need.

Do pregnant women actually obtain the recommended 2.6 milligrams of B_6 from their diet? Evidently, most women consume far less. A dietary survey of 57 pregnant women showed an average dietary intake of only 1.37 milligrams of B_6,[2] or little more than half the RDA. Seventy-seven percent of these women consumed less than two-thirds of the RDA, and 88 percent did not meet the RDA for B_6. Although this survey was performed on low-income women whose diets might have been of marginal quality, the findings were not much different from those obtained in other studies.[3] Clearly, many pregnant women need to supplement their diet with B_6.

There is also good reason to believe that many pregnant women need far more B_6 than 2.6 milligrams. Studies have shown that biochemical evidence of B_6 deficiency is relatively common during pregnancy. As much as 20 milligrams a day was needed by some women to correct this deficiency. Further, the studies showed that failure to correct B_6 deficiency during pregnancy may lead to complications, either for the mother or for the child.

As early as 1952, Max Wachstein, M.D., used a tryptophan load test (see chapter 1) and found that pregnant women excreted unusually large amounts of xanthurenic acid in their urine after ingesting a test dose of tryptophan.[4] This abnormal tryptophan metabolism suggested a vitamin B_6 deficiency. After the women took B_6 supplements (25 milligrams a day for six days), xanthurenic acid excretion returned to normal.

Since an abnormal tryptophan load test does not provide firm proof of B_6 deficiency, Dr. Wachstein confirmed his suspicion by testing B_6 levels another way.[5] A single 25-milligram dose of this vitamin was given to each of 56 pregnant women. The urinary excretion of 4-pyridoxic acid, the main metabolic end product of vitamin B_6, was then measured. In this test, a low excretion rate indicates a B_6 deficiency. Dr. Wachstein found that pregnant women excreted less of this B_6 metabolite than did other women. His earlier work suggesting that B_6 deficiency occurs in pregnancy was therefore confirmed.

Dr. Wachstein's studies were followed up by David B. Coursin, M.D., and his colleagues in 1961. Dr. Coursin measured blood levels of vitamin B_6 in 220 women during the course of normal pregnancy. There was little change during the first month, but after that there was a gradual and steady decline in B_6 levels. This vitamin is present in several forms in the blood (pyridoxamine phosphate, pyridoxal phosphate and pyridoxic acid). The concentration of pyridoxamine phosphate declined steadily during pregnancy, while that of the other two compounds fluctuated. There was a definite drop in the total concentration of B_6 molecules from the beginning to the end of pregnancy, however. Dr. Coursin found that a daily supplement of 6 milligrams of pyridoxine was not enough to prevent this decline in B_6 levels. It appeared that between 15 and 20 milligrams a day were necessary to keep B_6 levels at the same level they were at the start of pregnancy.[6]

More recent investigations by a group of Austrian doctors have also confirmed that B_6 deficiency may occur during pregnancy.[7] Pyridoxal phosphate concentrations were measured in the blood serum of 16 healthy pregnant women. These levels declined gradually and steadily throughout pregnancy. The largest drop occurred between the fourth and eighth months, corresponding to the period of greatest growth of the fetus. It appeared that the deficiency was due mainly to the transport of B_6 from the mother to the growing fetus.

According to the results of this study, the amount of B_6 the mother consumed correlated with the birth weight of her baby. Mothers who consumed less B_6 gave birth to smaller babies. This observation supported the results of a previous study by the same doctors. That study found that mothers who took supplements gave birth to significantly heavier babies than did other mothers. The effect of vitamin B_6 supplements on birth weight may be important, because low-birth-weight babies have a higher than normal incidence of brain damage at one year of age.

Scientists at the National Institute of Nutrition in India have also found that B_6 deficiency occurs frequently in pregnant women.[8] Sixteen women from a low socioeconomic group were studied in their third trimester. Ten of the women had skin lesions around the mouth, such as glossitis (inflammation of the tongue) or angular stomatitis (inflammation of the mucous membranes at the corners of the mouth). The other six women had normal skin. All 16 women had abnormal tryptophan metabolism as well as other biochemical evidence of B_6 deficiency. These abnormalities were more pronounced in women with oral lesions. Treatment with 25 milligrams of B_6 daily for five days cured the skin lesions and also corrected the abnormalities of tryptophan metabolism.

Thus, there is extensive documentation that vitamin B_6 deficiency occurs in pregnant women who do not take B_6 supplements. Still, the Committee on Dietary Allowances was not convinced that pregnant women need to take more than 2.6 milligrams of B_6 daily. "In spite of these observed alterations in laboratory indices," they concluded, "clinical evidence that vitamin B_6 deficiency is related to pregnancy complications is limited. Clinical trials of routine pyridoxine supplementation in pregnancy have failed to indicate any difference in outcome, casting doubt on any [preventive] or therapeutic benefit of the practice."[9]

To support their opinion, the committee cited a 1963 study by Robert W. Hillman, M.D., and co-workers.[10] Dr. Hillman studied the effect of B_6 supplements (20 milligrams a day) in 956 pregnant women. Compared with a group of 576 women who were given a placebo, there was no statistically significant difference in the incidence of pregnancy complications, such as toxemia, low birth weight, prematurity, etc. Dr. Hillman concluded that his results "do not provide support for a hypothesis that the routine administration of pyridoxine supplements to [pregnant] women produces a more favorable outcome of pregnancy."

Dr. Hillman's conclusion ignores two important observations. First, he found that the women taking B_6 reported "poor appetite" significantly less often than those receiving the placebo. Given the importance of good nutrition for the health of mother and child, improvement of appetite should hardly be considered a trivial effect of B_6 supplements. A second beneficial effect of B_6 supplements was a reduced incidence of dental cavities. Dr. Hillman reported this observation in a separate paper[11] and mentioned it in passing in the study cited by the committee.

If all that B_6 did were reduce the frequency of cavities, increase appetite and increase the birth weight of the infant, then supplementation would still be worthwhile, *especially, in view of the evidence that pregnant women are deficient in* B_6.

Reducing Pregnancy's Complications

Other reports suggest that vitamin B_6 supplements may be effective in the prevention or treatment of nausea and vomiting of pregnancy, toxemia and gestational diabetes. In addition, animal experiments have shown that adequate amounts of B_6 are necessary to promote normal brain development and to prevent some birth defects.

In their review of the data, the committee ignored all this research. They also presented a rather biased interpretation of Dr. Hillman's study. In the first place, they referred to his work as "clinical trials." There was only one clinical trial, not several—which yielded negative results. It was misleading for the committee to suggest that Dr. Hillman's work had been confirmed by others, particularly since they had ignored research that contradicted his findings.

It was also misleading of the committee to state that Dr. Hillman's work "cast doubt" on the value of B_6. The correct statement would have been that the study *did not prove* B_6 prevented complications of pregnancy. Failure to prove that the vitamin works is not the same as showing that it does not work. Dr. Hillman recognized this in discussing his results.[10] He stated: "A larger sample size also might yield statistically significant differences between groups receiving supplements and those not receiving supplements of pyridoxine." Dr. Hillman did not report the number of women who suffered the various complications of pregnancy (except for toxemia). He merely stated that there were no significant differences between B_6 and a placebo. His statement about a larger sample size suggests that there may have been some trends in favor of the vitamin. In other words, the B_6 group may have fared better than the placebo group with respect to complications of pregnancy, but the differences were not statistically significant. As I will explain in chapter 5, lack of statistical significance simply means we are less than 95 percent certain that B_6 prevents complications of pregnancy. It still might be beneficial, but we would need to study a larger number of women in order to prove this. In the past several years it has become clear that doctors have often erroneously rejected potentially valuable therapies because they do not understand the meaning of statistical significance.

In view of the evidence presented in this chapter and the studies showing that B_6 deficiency is common in pregnancy, the conclusion of the committee is untenable. In fact, it seems reasonable to suggest that nearly all pregnant women should be receiving at least 10 to 20 milligrams of B_6 every day. Since the most that can be obtained from a good diet is about 2 to 5 milligrams, supplements are clearly necessary. There is evidence that B_6 supplements are of value for each of the following complications of pregnancy.

Nausea and Vomiting

As many as 50 percent of women experience nausea and vomiting during the first trimester of pregnancy. These symptoms may range from mild morning sickness to vomiting so severe that it requires hospitalization and intravenous feeding. When vomiting becomes severe, it is called hyperemesis gravidarum, or pernicious vomiting of pregnancy. The cause of nausea and vomiting is unknown, but it is believed to be related to changes in hormone levels. The anxiety and tension that accompany some pregnancies may also contribute to these symptoms.

Some mild cases of morning sickness will respond to changes in diet. Women are often advised to eat some crackers immediately upon awakening and then to go back to bed for 20 minutes. After that, they should get up and eat breakfast. Eating small, frequent meals during the day may also help. These conservative measures, however, do not always eliminate the problem. Some doctors may prescribe sedatives such as phenobarbital or antinausea medications such as Bendectin. Until the spring of 1983, Bendectin was being taken by as many as 25 percent of all pregnant women in the United States.

On June 9, 1983, Merrell Dow Pharmaceuticals sent a Mailgram to American physicians to inform them that the company had "reluctantly decided to cease production of Bendectin." Articles published in the *National Enquirer* and elsewhere had alleged that this drug caused birth defects in the infants of mothers who took it. There was actually very little scientific evidence suggesting that Bendectin was dangerous,[12] but, because of the publicity, hundreds of parents sued Merrell Dow, alledging that Bendectin had caused them to give birth to a deformed child. As the cost of defending itself against lawsuits became intolerable

(Merrell Dow lost one $750,000 judgment, which was later overturned), the company felt it had no choice but to remove Bendectin from the market.

After this decision was announced, the American College of Obstetrics and Gynecology quickly released a statement lamenting the "significant therapeutic gap" that had been created by the loss of this drug. Bendectin had been the only drug approved by the Food and Drug Administration for morning sickness. Without the drug, the obstetricians claimed, millions of women would be denied relief from this common complication of pregnancy.

In reality, there was little reason for doctors to be so concerned about the removal of Bendectin from the market. Evidence over the past 40 years had shown that vitamin B_6 is also useful for nausea and vomiting of pregnancy. In fact, Bendectin contains 10 milligrams of B_6 per capsule, and at least one study has suggested that the vitamin is the active ingredient in Bendectin.

The beneficial effect of B_6 on the nausea and vomiting of pregnancy was reported as long ago as 1942[13]. Raymond S. Willis and colleagues at the Department of Obstetrics, Baylor University College of Medicine, administered intravenous or intramuscular injections of vitamin B_6 to 37 women and found that most of them experienced improvement or complete relief from their nausea and vomiting. They also gave thiamine (vitamin B_1) injections to a number of women, but felt that B_6 worked better.

The following year, other physicians confirmed these results.[14] Complete relief was obtained in 38 of 40 women treated with intravenous injections of 25 or 50 milligrams of B_6. Oral doses of 30 to 60 milligrams were not helpful. Improvement usually occurred within 6 to 24 hours after the first injection. Twenty-two patients experienced complete and permanent relief after the first injection. In others, the symptoms eventually returned, but repeat injections of B_6 were again effective. Interestingly, six patients with seborrheic dermatitis noted great improvement in their skin after they received the B_6.

Stimulated by these studies, B. Bernard Weinstein, M.D., and associates at Tulane University began studying B_6[15] and reported their results in 1944. They treated 78 women with oral B_6 in daily doses ranging from 30 to 80 milligrams. Women whose vomiting was so severe that they couldn't keep down any food were first given the vitamin by injection (100 milligrams a day). When the vomiting was controlled, they were given B_6 by mouth. Complete or considerable relief was obtained in nearly all cases, usually within one to three days. Of the ten patients with the most severe nausea and vomiting, eight lost their symptoms entirely after this treatment. The authors were particularly gratified by the results in these severe cases, since patients with these symptoms occasionally require hospitalization and intravenous feeding.

The beneficial effect of B_6 was also confirmed in a more recent study.[16] Twenty pregnant women with hyperemesis gravidarum were treated with 200 milligrams of B_6 daily. Their symptoms cleared up rapidly. Before treatment with B_6, the level of pyridoxal phosphate in the blood serum was significantly lower in the women with hyperemesis than in other women at the same stage of pregnancy. The low levels of B_6 may, of course, have been due to the vomiting. On the other hand, B_6 deficiency could have been a cause of the symptoms.

One investigator, H. Close Hesseltine, M.D., failed to find any benefits from B_6.[17] Sixteen patients with nausea and vomiting were treated with either pyridoxine (100 milligrams daily by mouth and 100 milligrams intramuscularly twice a week) or placebo. The vitamin produced no better results than placebo treatment. Only 3 of 11 patients treated first with the vitamin had good results. Dr. Hesseltine suggested that previously reported beneficial effects of B_6 may have actually been a placebo effect. Nausea and vomiting of pregnancy is known to improve frequently after treatment with a placebo. In none of the other studies was the effect of B_6 compared to that of a placebo. Dr. Hesseltine also pointed out that nausea and vomiting usually disappear after the third month of pregnancy. He suggested that many of the improvements attributed to vitamin treatment were actually spontaneous remissions. Dr. Hesseltine also criticized previous investigators for using several treatments at once. For example, in some studies, sedatives were prescribed and dietary advice was given in addition to B_6 supplements, so it was impossible to tell if the studies' results were due to these other treatments.

Dr. Hesseltine did raise some important issues; however, his criticisms were not entirely valid. In one of the studies, for example, the doctors made a point not to prescribe sedatives or recommend dietary changes, yet the results from B_6 were still excellent. In addition, the rapid relief of symptoms from B_6 therapy makes it unlikely that improvement was due to spontaneous remission. Several different groups noticed that symptoms improved within 6 to 72 hours after treatment was begun. Spontaneous remission, on the other hand, usually occurs only at the end of the third month of pregnancy. It is difficult to believe that so many women would have sought treatment just at the time their symptoms were about to go away.

The possibility of a placebo response cannot be ruled out. In one study, the majority of women did respond to a placebo. On the other hand, some of the results suggest that the benefits from B₆ were real. Some women who had failed to respond to other treatments improved rapidly after taking B₆. If these women were "placebo responders," then they probably would have benefited from the earlier treatments. In one study, B₆ cured eight of ten women who probably would have had to be hospitalized otherwise. If that was a placebo effect, then we should have more of such placebos.

It is not clear why Dr. Hesseltine's results differed from those of so many other doctors. The fact that only 3 of 11 B₆-treated patients got good results was somewhat peculiar. Even placebo therapy has been known to produce better results than that. Dr. Hesseltine remarked that he was surprised that other doctors had found so many women with nausea and vomiting in such a short time. In his experience, these symptoms were rarely severe enough to require treatment in pregnant women. It seems that Dr. Hesseltine may have accepted only the more severe cases for his study of B₆. Perhaps, because of vomiting, his patients were not retaining the oral dose. The twice-a-week injections might therefore not have been frequent enough to produce results. Some of the investigators who observed good results in severe cases had given daily injections until the vomiting was controlled.

Today the standard opinion about B₆ is that it does not work for nausea and vomiting of pregnancy. The third edition of the *AMA Drug Evaluations* states: "Pyridoxine hydrochloride (vitamin B₆) has been used in the management of nausea and vomiting of pregnancy, but it is in-effective."[18] It is hard to understand how the AMA group could come to such a conclusion from the available data. The most recent edition of a standard nutrition textbook presents a more accurate picture. It states: "Pyridoxine has been used for a number of years by obstetricians for the control of nausea and vomiting of pregnancy. The effectiveness of this treatment has not been proven by carefully controlled studies."[19] Given enough research interest and funding, we may eventually deter-mine, once and for all, whether B₆ is effective for nausea and vomiting of pregnancy.

One study comparing B₆ to a prescription drug indicated that B₆ relieves nausea and vomiting of pregnancy in 75 percent of women tested.[20] If it turns out that B₆ is nothing more than a placebo, then so be it. Some ailments respond well to placebos. Laboratory studies suggest that pregnant women should be taking B_6 supplements anyway. In cases where a placebo is the treatment of choice, doctors should learn to prescribe safe ones.

In the meantime, the use of B_6 for this purpose should not be discouraged. To reduce the risk of damage to the fetus, pregnant women should try to avoid taking drugs whenever possible.

Toxemia of Pregnancy

One of the most serious complications of pregnancy is known as toxemia. This disorder is a metabolic disturbance that occurs only during pregnancy. It is characterized by high blood pressure, edema (swelling) and proteinuria (excretion of protein in the urine). In some cases, if it goes untreated, toxemia may progress to convulsions, coma and death. Every year, hundreds of mothers and more than 30,000 infants die as a direct result of toxemia.[21]

Acute toxemia of pregnancy occurs in two forms: toxemia in its nonconvulsive form is called preeclampsia. When convulsions and coma occur, the condition is called eclampsia. The cause of toxemia is not known. We do know, however, that it is a disease of civilization and that women of low socioeconomic status are at increased risk. Perhaps poor nutrition is a contributing factor in these women.

Toxemia occurs in about 6 to 7 percent of all pregnant women. Signs of this problem usually begin around the sixth or seventh month and disappear promptly after delivery. The classic manifestations are swelling (especially in the hands and legs), high blood pressure and loss of protein in the urine. Every attempt should be made to treat the illness at this stage, before it progresses and becomes serious. Common recommendations for early preeclampsia include bed rest, sedatives, low-salt diet and diuretics. The use of diuretics and low-salt diets is controversial, however. Many physicians believe these treatments aggravate the problem. There is some evidence that increasing dietary protein may reduce the incidence of this disorder. Other nutritional deficiencies should also be corrected.

If symptoms progress to the point where convulsions seem imminent, a doctor administers large doses of intravenous magnesium. This mineral lowers blood pressure and decreases the tendency for seizures to occur. In large doses, however, magnesium can also be toxic, so it must be given with caution.

There is evidence that vitamin B$_6$ plays a role in both the prevention and treatment of this obstetrical catastrophe. The concentration of pyridoxal phosphate, the active form of vitamin B$_6$, was measured in placental tissue of a series of pregnant women.[21] Women who had suffered preeclampsia had markedly lower levels of this vitamin than those who had had a normal pregnancy. It is possible that a deficiency of B$_6$ might have altered the function of the placenta and somehow contributed to the development of toxemia.

Of course, the presence of low B$_6$ levels alone does not prove cause and effect. B$_6$ deficiency could have been a result of the toxemia, or simply an unrelated finding. Hoping to determine whether B$_6$ deficiency is really a cause of preeclampsia, Dr. Wachstein and Louis W. Graffeo, M.D., studied 820 pregnant middle-income women.[22] Half these women were given tablets containing 10 milligrams of pyridoxine in addition to multivitamins. The other half took multivitamins but no extra B$_6$. Women who had received the B$_6$ had a significantly lower incidence of preeclampsia than the control group. In the experimental group, only 1.7 percent of the women developed this complication. In the control group, the figure was 4.4 percent. The study by Drs. Wachstein and Graffeo strongly suggested that vitamin B$_6$ deficiency is a cause of toxemia of pregnancy.

Dr. Hillman, whose work was discussed earlier, could not confirm the results of Drs. Wachstein and Graffeo.[10] In Dr. Hillman's study, women received a multivitamin with or without 20 milligrams of B$_6$ along with placebo lozenges. A third group took multivitamins lacking B$_6$, but took 20 milligrams of B$_6$ in lozenge form. There was no significant reduction in the incidence of preeclampsia in women who received B$_6$. In fact, the B$_6$ groups had a somewhat higher incidence (3.0 to 3.6 percent) than the group that received no B$_6$ (2.1 percent). The discrepancy in results between these two studies might be related to the fact that different socioeconomic classes were studied. The women who apparently benefited from B$_6$ supplements were middle class. Those who did not benefit were of low socioeconomic status. Exactly how this difference might affect the results is unclear, however.

Perhaps the most exciting work on vitamin B$_6$ and toxemia of pregnancy has been done by John M. Ellis, M.D., a family doctor from

Mount Pleasant, Texas. Dr. Ellis became interested in vitamin B_6 in 1961 and has been using it extensively in his practice ever since. In his 1973 book *Vitamin B_6: The Doctor's Report*,[23] he detailed the dramatic results he has achieved using high doses of B_6 for a wide range of medical problems.

At the time his book was published in 1973, Dr. Ellis had treated 225 pregnant women with large doses of vitamin B_6. From this series of cases, he reached the conclusion that nearly all cases of edema of pregnancy could be controlled or prevented by vitamin B_6. Some women responded to 50 milligrams a day. Others required as much as 450 milligrams a day before the edema disappeared. Occasionally, injections of the vitamin were necessary to bring about an improvement in the edema. Only 6 women out of the 225 failed to respond to vitamin B_6. These results were achieved *even though none of the women were given diuretics or told to restrict their salt*. Dr. Ellis observed repeatedly that the 10 milligrams of B_6 present in some prenatal vitamin tablets was insufficient to prevent edema. On the other hand, some women with marked edema lost between 10 and 15 pounds of water weight within two weeks, when given between 50 and 450 milligrams of B_6 daily. (That level of B_6 should be taken only under your doctor's supervision.)

Dr. Ellis's observations have important implications. Edema is present in about one-third of all pregnant women in the United States. Edema is a cause of concern to obstetricians because it may represent an early warning sign of toxemia. If large doses of B_6 can control the edema, then they might conceivably prevent the development of more-severe signs of toxemia as well.

Remember, B_6 treatment eliminated the need for salt restriction and diuretics. This observation is important. Many physicians become nervous when edema appears. They prescribe diuretics and restrict salt intake in the hope of preventing toxemia. Most doctors today believe that these practices are dangerous, however. Diuretics tend to make the blood more concentrated, which might restrict circulation to the fetus. Salt deficiency may also impair normal fetal development. If doctors followed the lead of Dr. Ellis and began using B_6 for edema, then they would no doubt be less tempted to prescribe diuretics and restrict sodium intake.

Dr. Ellis strongly believed that all women should receive at least 50 milligrams of B_6 daily throughout pregnancy. Many will require considerably more than that. In addition, Dr. Ellis recommended that all women should take at least 500 milligrams of magnesium daily. Magnesium also seems to inhibit the development of toxemia, and this mineral works in conjunction with B_6 in a number of different ways.

It would be interesting to speculate on why Dr. Hillman's study did not show a protective effect of B_6 against toxemia. Perhaps his subjects were malnourished and needed far more B_6 than the 20 milligrams they were getting each day. It would be worthwhile to repeat Dr. Hillman's study using 50 milligrams of pyridoxine.

It might be hard to believe that some women would need almost 200 times the RDA for vitamin B_6 in order to make it through their pregnancy in good health; however, that is what Dr. Ellis repeatedly observed. Since toxemia is a disease of civilization—it occurs in a society bombarded with foods and chemicals that interfere with vitamin B_6 metabolism—it should not be surprising that the added stress imposed by a growing fetus on its mother's B_6 reserves might throw some women into a state of marked deficiency.

Dr. Ellis also found that other symptoms in pregnant women responded to B_6 supplements. These include numbness, tingling and loss of sensation in the fingertips, weakness of hand grip, impaired flexion of the fingers, pain in the finger joints and nocturnal paralysis of the arm. He also observed that severe muscle spasms in the legs and feet were improved or completely relieved with 50 to 450 milligrams of B_6 daily. Muscle spasms in pregnancy are usually thought to be due to calcium deficiency. In many cases, the spasms are indeed eliminated by calcium supplements.[24] In others, however, calcium is ineffective. Dr. Ellis found that women who had not responded to calcium supplements were relieved by taking B_6.

Pregnant women should be cautious about putting any substance in their body, even vitamins. Are large doses of B_6 safe? Dr. Ellis did not observe any obvious side effects from daily doses of 50 to 450 milligrams throughout pregnancy. In addition, he found that as much as 1,000 milligrams could be given daily for several days without toxicity. These large doses did not appear to increase the need for B_6 in the infants after birth. Although B_6 as prescribed by Dr. Ellis does appear to be safe, this vitamin should not be used indiscriminately. It should certainly not be taken in large amounts without the supervision of an obstetrician. To ensure a margin of safety, the lowest effective dose should be used. If the pregnant women eliminates food additives from her diet, emphasizes foods grown without the use of chemicals and avoids processed fats, then she may be able to get by with considerably less B_6.

Magnesium and zinc should also be given in conjunction with B_6, since both of these minerals work together with this important vitamin. Deficiencies of both zinc[25] and magnesium[26] are not uncommon in pregnant women. Not only do these minerals interact with B_6, but they are also important in their own right. Animal studies suggest that even moderate zinc deficiency may cause abnormalities in the offspring.[27] In addition, magnesium deficiency has been associated with spontaneous abortions.[28]

Gestational Diabetes

Abnormal carbohydrate metabolism occasionally occurs in pregnant women. Apparently, the stress of pregnancy hinders glucose tolerance (the ability to regulate blood sugar) in some women. The term "gestational diabetes" is used to describe abnormal glucose tolerance in a pregnant woman who has no other signs or symptoms of diabetes. Although some women with gestational diabetes develop true diabetes later in life, more often than not the problem disappears within six weeks after delivery. Nevertheless, it is becoming increasingly clear that gestational diabetes should be identified and treated. Even if this disorder is mild, it may, when untreated, increase the risk of death in the newborn.

The usual management of gestational diabetes includes dietary changes and, when necessary, small doses of insulin. There is also evidence that vitamin B_6 supplements may be useful for some women with this problem. In 1975 doctors from the Netherlands studied the effect of B_6 supplements on 14 women with gestational diabetes. Prior to treatment, 13 of these women excreted increased amounts of xanthurenic acid in their urine during a tryptophan load test. This finding suggested a B_6 deficiency. All patients were put on a diet and were given 100 milligrams of pyridoxine daily for two weeks. At that time, a repeat test showed no evidence of B_6 deficiency. Further, the women's glucose tolerance improved after two weeks of B_6 therapy. Twelve of the 14 patients no longer had evidence of gestational diabetes. It is possible that the change in diet may have contributed to the improvement; however, since previous experience showed that dietary measures alone had a negligible effect on glucose tolerance, the researchers concluded that the beneficial changes were due to the B_6 supplements.[29]

Because of the importance of these findings, other doctors soon attempted to confirm the work of the Dutch doctors. W. N. Spellacy, M.D., and colleagues performed an intravenous glucose tolerance test on 13 women with gestational diabetes. The test was repeated after two weeks' treatment with B_6 (100 milligrams a day). Glucose tolerance improved significantly after B_6 therapy[30] without a rise in plasma insulin levels. According to Dr. Spellacy, these results "suggest that the vitamin B_6 treatment increased the plasma insulin's biologic activity." In other words, B_6 appeared to make the body's available insulin more effective, rather than stimulating production of more insulin.

Other investigators were unable to find a beneficial effect of B_6 in gestational diabetes. Richard P. Perkins, M.D., treated four women with B_6 (100 milligrams daily) for three weeks. No improvement in glucose tolerance occurred in any of the four patients.[31] In another study, performed in South Africa,[32] 13 women with gestational diabetes were found to excrete excessive amounts of xanthurenic acid after a tryptophan load, suggesting vitamin B_6 deficiency. These women were then given 100 milligrams of B_6 daily for 14 to 23 days. Although the abnormal tryptophan metabolism was corrected by B_6 treatment, glucose tolerance improved in only 2 of the 13 women.

There are two possible explanations for the contradictory findings in these studies. One possibility is that improvements thought to be due to B_6 therapy were actually due to dietary changes. Another is that in the Dutch study, the women remained at home and were followed up at an outpatient clinic. In the South African study, the women were admitted to the hospital and stayed there until they delivered. The hospitalized women were probably much less active than the outpatients. Physical activity is one factor known to improve glucose tolerance. It is possible, therefore, that B_6 therapy had indeed helped the South African patients, but that this benefit was counterbalanced by a sedentary existence.

The possibility that B_6 might help gestational diabetes is exciting. At this time, however, the evidence is contradictory. A larger, placebo-controlled study of perhaps 100 women might provide a more definitive answer about whether B_6 is effective. In the meantime, obstetricians who choose to prescribe B_6 for gestational diabetes should not be chastised. The use of B_6 during pregnancy appears to be quite safe.

Further discussion on the nutritional management of diabetes is presented in chapter 9.

Effects on the Infant

A deficiency of vitamin B_6 during pregnancy, aside from adversely affecting the mother's health, may also lead to negative consequences for the child. This vitamin is necessary for normal brain development. When pregnant rats were fed a diet low in B_6, their offspring showed gross neurological symptoms shortly after birth.[33]

In addition, B_6 deficiency may be a contributing factor in the development of birth defects. In a recent study, pregnant mice were injected with cortisone to produce cleft palate in their offspring. Sixty-eight percent of the offspring of these cortisone-treated mothers developed this birth defect. When the mothers were also given additional vitamin B_6 in their diet, the incidence of cleft palate fell to 26 percent, however.[34]

These findings may be relevant to the problem of cleft palate in humans. Some women must take cortisonelike drugs during pregnancy, because of a chronic illness. Vitamin B_6 supplements might reduce the incidence of cleft palate in infants of these women. The cause of cleft palate in humans is not known, but the results of this animal study suggest that the possible influence of B_6 deficiency should be examined more closely.

In another study, pregnant rats were given a B_6-deficient diet and a B_6 antagonist, 4-deoxypyridoxine. Their fetuses were small and appeared anemic. Major fetal malformations included cleft palate, omphalocele (a protrusion of the intestines through a defect in the navel), exencephaly (a defect in development of the skull), micrognathia (abnormally small jaws), defects in the fingers, and improper development of the spleen.[35]

The effects of maternal deficiency of B_6 on human offspring has been less well documented; however, there is some indication that it may be a problem. In one study, the mother's vitamin B_6 intake was found to be related to her infant's Apgar score. The Apgar score is a standard measurement of distress in the newborn infant. Five criteria are taken into account: the newborn's skin coloring, ability to cry, heart rate, respiratory effort and muscle tone. The score ranges from one to ten. Any score below seven is considered evidence of distress, probably due to inadequate oxygen supply. There is a close relationship between a low Apgar score five minutes after birth and the incidence of brain damage at one year of age. Dietary intake of vitamin B_6 was estimated in 106 pregnant women by means of a three-day diet record. Mothers whose infants had unsatisfactory Apgar scores (less than seven) one minute after birth had significantly lower B_6 intakes than mothers whose infants had satisfactory scores (greater than or equal to seven).[36] The Apgar score at one minute is not as closely associated with brain damage as is the five-minute score. Nevertheless, there is some association between one-minute Apgar scores and subsequent neurologic problems. This study therefore suggests that low maternal B_6 intake may increase the risk of brain damage in the child. Of course, other characteristics in these women may also have been important. For example, the women with low B_6 intake may have also consumed less of other key nutrients. Exactly how much B_6 deficiency contributed to the low Apgar scores is therefore not known. In view of the animal studies demonstrating the importance of B_6, however, supplementation with this nutrient seems advisable for all pregnant women.

As mentioned above, Dr. Hillman did not find any difference in pregnancy outcome from the addition of 20 milligrams of B_6 to the mother's diet. On the other hand, he did not assess the neurologic status of the infants at one year of age. Perhaps he would have noticed an effect of B_6 if he had done so. It is known that low Apgar scores and low birth weights both increase the risk of brain damage at one year. The evidence shows that B_6 supplements are associated with an increase in both Apgar score and birth weight. Dr. Hillman recognized that his study may have failed to detect some subtle effects of B_6 supplementation. "Conceivably," he wrote, "The criteria employed in this study are too conventional and too crude to permit identification of more subtle, but possibly more meaningful clinical effects."[10] Unfortunately, the Committee on Dietary Allowances was less open-minded about the possibility that B_6 supplements might be necessary for pregnant women.

Further information on the association between B_6 and brain damage came from a study of the offspring of toxemic women. The blood plasma level of B_6 was measured in these infants and found to be significantly lower than that of the offspring of normal pregnancies.[37] Children of toxemic mothers are known to have a much higher than normal incidence of mental retardation. Perhaps a deficiency of B_6 at birth is responsible for impaired brain development and subsequent retardation. When preeclamptic mothers were given vitamin B_6 before delivery, the infants did not have any evidence of deficiency at birth. Thus, B_6 supplementation of toxemic mothers may not only improve the condition of the mother but may also increase the chances the child will develop normally.

Deficiency in Cigarette Smokers

Vitamin B_6 levels were assessed in a group of pregnant smokers. Despite intakes of B_6 similar to nonsmoking pregnant women, the smokers had significantly lower plasma levels of the vitamin. Enzyme stimulation studies showed that 49 percent of smokers, but only 23 percent of nonsmokers, had evidence of B_6 deficiency.[38] Average birth weight of the infants of smokers was about 300 grams less than for infants of nonsmokers. Some of the growth retardation due to smoking was prevented when the mothers increased their intake of B_6 during pregnancy, however. This study demonstrated that cigarette smoking adversely affects the level of vitamin B_6 in the body. Pregnant women should not smoke, but those who feel they must smoke should be sure to increase their vitamin B_6 intake.

The presence of B_6 antagonists in tobacco smoke may explain the adverse effect of cigarette smoking on B_6. Hydrazine, found in both tobacco and tobacco smoke,[39] is known to be a potent inhibitor of vitamin B_6 metabolism. Initially this chemical was assumed to be a breakdown product of maleic hydrazide, which is sprayed on tobacco plants to prevent sprouting. Hydrazine was later discovered to be present naturally in tobacco. The chemical structure of maleic hydrazide suggests that it, too, may be a B_6 antagonist.

Suppressing Lactation

The level of vitamin B_6 in a mother's body relates directly to the amount of B_6 in her breast milk. The Committee on Dietary Allowances has suggested that a daily intake of 2.5 milligrams of B_6 during lactation will provide a level of B_6 in the milk adequate to meet an infant's needs.[9]

Although nursing is advisable for a number of reasons, some women are unable to breast-feed their baby. In these women, milk production must be somehow shut off, or else painful engorgement of the breasts will occur. It appears that B_6 supplements may be capable of suppressing lactation. In one study, 100 women were given 200 milligrams of B_6

three times a day, beginning on the second or third day after delivery. Treatment was continued for six days. Lactation was successfully suppressed in 95 percent of the women within one week, compared with 83 percent treated with stilbestrol and 17 percent of those given a placebo.[40] In another study, however, vitamin B_6 supplements failed to suppress lactation in 14 women.[41] Since the conditions under which B_6 suppresses lactation are unclear, women who wish to nurse should be careful not to take massive amounts of this vitamin. Large doses in the range of 600 milligrams a day may indeed shut off the milk supply. We don't know exactly how much B_6 is safe in this respect. I have used 50 milligrams of B_6 daily for various reasons in several nursing mothers. None of them had any problems with nursing. No one has reported an effect of B_6 on lactation at doses less than 600 milligrams a day. Still, nursing women should be careful, and they should take B_6 only under the supervision of a physician.

There is considerable evidence that vitamin B_6 deficiency is a common occurrence in pregnant women. This deficiency may arise from hormonal changes, from the nutritional demands of the fetus and from dietary and environmental factors that promote B_6 deficiency. Vitamin B_6 may be of value in the prevention and treatment of nausea and vomiting of pregnancy, toxemia and gestational diabetes. In addition, this vitamin may help prevent birth defects and brain damage in infants. The exact B_6 requirement is not known and probably varies greatly, depending on the woman. It seems clear, however, that the RDA of 2.6 milligrams a day is far too low. There is evidence that most pregnant women should be receiving at least 10 to 20 milligrams of B_6 a day. Some may need considerably more. In any case, massive amounts of B_6 should not be taken by mothers who wish to nurse.

Part III

Better Moods and Behavior

Chapter
Depression 4

Depression is the nation's most common emotional disorder, affecting approximately 25 percent of all Americans at one time or another over a lifetime. The National Institute of Mental Health has estimated that about 20 million Americans, or as many as 13 percent of adults, may be suffering from serious depression at any given time,[1] and depression is the leading cause of hospital admissions for mental illness.

Depression causes untold suffering for its victims and their families, lowers productivity and burdens society with enormous medical expenses. Its greatest toll, however, is the high suicide rate. According to the *Statistical Abstract of the United States*, there were more than 27,000 suicides in the United States in 1979.[2] This number is probably greatly underestimated, since many deaths reported as automobile accidents were probably unreported suicides.

Although drugs provide relief in many cases, as many as 30 percent of depressed individuals fail to respond to the best that modern medicine has to offer. Further, despite advances in psychiatric treatment, both depression and suicide seem to be increasing.

Depressed people may suffer from any of a wide range of physical and emotional complaints. Common symptoms include insomnia, changes in appetite, digestive disturbances, weight loss, loss of sex drive and feelings of inadequacy. Depressed people tend to feel hopeless, apathetic and unable to experience pleasure. They may feel guilty, sluggish,

58

apprehensive and have premonitions of impending disaster. Often they lose their self-esteem regardless of their true abilities: A research scientist might come to see himself as stupid, or an accomplished musician might become convinced she lacks talent. Depressed people also tend to develop a large assortment of aches and pains, and many become alcoholics.

Depression can be classified into two major categories: reactive and endogenous. Reactive depression arises from some situations, such as financial difficulties, marital problems or death of a loved one. People who suffer from this type of depression often improve with time or with the insights that come from psychotherapy.

In cases where no obvious event can be said to have triggered the illness, the depression is labeled "endogenous" because it appears to come from inside the person. People who suffer from endogenous depression often fail to respond to psychotherapy and are incapable of lifting themselves out of their misery. Their depression may linger or worsen to the point where they become unable to function.

The Link with Brain Biochemistry

Research during the past three decades has linked depression to certain abnormalities of brain biochemistry. It now appears that depression (particularly the endogenous type) is often a biochemical disorder rather than a purely psychological illness. Of course, psychological and biochemical factors may interact. For example, a person may have a mild biochemical imbalance in the brain that produces a few chronic but mild symptoms of depression. This person would probably have no major emotional difficulty unless a life crisis threw him into a state of severe depression. Other people become depressed even though they are apparently satisfied with the way their life is going. In these cases the depression is often caused solely by abnormal brain biochemistry. When the metabolic abnormality is discovered and properly treated, the depression often disappears, even without any attempts at psychotherapy or counseling.

I want to emphasize that there are many different causes of biochemical depression, and proper treatment varies from person to person. The brain's metabolism is extremely complex. Dozens of different molecules found in the brain are known to affect mood and behavior, and their interactions are complicated and poorly understood. Brain metabolism can go awry in countless ways, any number of which might trigger depression. As we shall see, some of these abnormalities, and the depression they produce, can be corrected by vitamin B_6.

The first indication that depression could be a biochemical disorder came in the 1950's,[3] when a few patients being treated for high blood pressure with a rauwolfia alkaloid (reserpine) developed depression. Around the same time, it was discovered that patients receiving the antituberculous drug iproniazid experienced unusual mood elevations. Further study revealed that these two drugs exerted opposite effects on the brain. Reserpine caused reduced brain levels of amines (including norepinephrine and serotonin). Treatment with iproniazid, on the other hand, led to an increase in the concentration of amines. These observations suggested that an increase in brain amines is associated with mood elevation, whereas depletion of these amines is related to depression, a concept strengthened when scientists discovered that some antidepressant drugs also increased amine levels in the brain.

Serotonin and norepinephrine function as neurotransmitters, "chemical messengers" that transmit information from one neuron (nerve cell) to the next. Neurotransmitters affect our mood, our behavior and our thoughts. These molecules are released from nerve endings into the spaces between neurons, called synapses. The neurotransmitter travels across the synapse and transmits its chemical message to the adjacent neuron. This message is then translated into an electrical signal that travels down the length of the second neuron. When this electrical signal reaches the other end, it triggers the release of more neurotransmitters into the next synapse. After the neurotransmitter has done its job, it is either pulled back inside the neuron to be reused or else it is broken down by enzymes. This chain reaction allows rapid transmission of nerve signals to any portion of the nervous system.

Apparently, a deficiency of neurotransmitter molecules can cause depression. Such a deficiency might occur in several ways: The brain may not manufacture adequate quantities of these molecules; the enzymes that break down the neurotransmitter might be overactive; or the neuron on the receiving end may have lost its ability to respond to the chemical message.

The Effects of Drugs

The class of drugs called tricyclic antidepressants (imipramine, amitriptyline, desipramine, etc.) works by preventing serotonin and norepinephrine from returning to the neuron that released them. Instead, these molecules remain in the synapse, where they transmit one signal after another, so each molecule does the work of several. Another series of antidepressant drugs is known as monoamine oxidase inhibitors. Most of the neurotransmitters are monoamines because they contain a single amine molecule. When an enzyme called monoamine oxidase oxidizes these amines, they become inactive. A monoamine oxidase inhibitor therefore allows the neurotransmitters to remain active longer.

Drug therapy is effective in as many as 70 percent of depressed people; however, antidepressants can also provoke a host of side effects. Tricyclic antidepressants may produce adverse cardiovascular reactions, including high blood pressure, rapid heartbeat, palpitations, abnormal heart rhythm, congestive heart failure and even heart attacks or strokes. They may also trigger various psychiatric reactions, such as confusion, hallucinations, disorientation, anxiety, insomnia and nightmares. Tricyclics may cause neurologic problems, such as numbness, tingling, loss of coordination and balance, seizures and ringing in the ears. They can also cause dry mouth, blurred vision, constipation, urinary retention, skin rashes, swelling, nausea, vomiting, impotence and changes in blood sugar levels. Patients may suffer nausea, headache and malaise if these drugs are discontinued abruptly after long-term use.

Monoamine oxidase inhibitors have reportedly caused some of the same side effects as tricyclics. In addition, they may produce a unique and serious side effect: hypertensive crisis—blood pressure so high that it may trigger bleeding inside the brain or even death. Severe hypertension can strike if a person taking one of these drugs also eats foods containing an amine called tyramine, such as aged cheese, wine, yogurt, liver, yeast extract, certain beans, caffeine and chocolate. One of the monoamine oxidase inhibitors is phenelzine sulfate (Nardil). As mentioned in chapter 1, this drug is a hydrazine molecule known to antagonize vitamin B_6. As we'll soon see, deficiency of this vitamin appears to be one cause of depression. It is therefore possible that prolonged use of Nardil could actually make some cases of depression worse. Fortunately, monoamine oxidase inhibitors are not used very often. Because of their potential for causing serious harm, they are usually reserved for cases where other antidepressants have failed.

Several new antidepressant medications have recently appeared on the market. Trazodone (Desyrel) and maprotiline hydrochloride (Ludiomil) cause cardiovascular toxicity less frequently than do older medications. Still, the list of potential side effects from these new drugs is disturbing. Although the development of tricyclic antidepressants has been a godsend for millions of victims of depression, the toxicity of these drugs makes them less than ideal therapy. Furthermore, about 30 percent of the time, tricyclics do not help very much.

During the past decade there has been a growing interest in the so-called "orthomolecular" treatment of psychiatric illness. The term "orthomolecular" means "the correct molecules." Professor Linus Pauling, a two-time Nobel Prize winner, coined this term in 1968. He defined orthomolecular psychiatry as "the treatment of mental disease by the provision of the optimum molecular environment for the mind, especially the optimum concentrations of substances normally present in the body."[4] The use of compounds already present in the body is usually considerably safer than drug therapy.

There are two distinct orthomolecular strategies for raising the level of brain amines. One strategy might be called precursor therapy. A precursor is a molecule that the body's enzymes convert into an active compound such as serotonin or norepinephrine. Each of these neurotransmitters has a precursor naturally present in the diet. Serotonin and norepinephrine are both synthesized from amino acids: serotonin from tryptophan and norepinephrine from tyrosine. Supplementation with these amino acids might therefore relieve the symptoms of depression by increasing neurotransmitter levels in the brain.

Clinical studies have shown that tryptophan and tyrosine do indeed have antidepressant activity. In some cases tryptophan has worked as well as the tricyclic antidepressant imipramine.[5] In a few cases tyrosine was found to be effective even after standard drugs had failed.[6]

It may seem more rational to treat depressed patients with the neurotransmitters themselves, rather than with their precursors. The use of neurotransmitters does not work, however, because of the "blood-brain barrier," a biochemical wall that prevents certain molecules in the bloodstream from entering the brain. Tryptophan and tyrosine can cross this barrier with little difficulty, whereas serotonin and norepinephrine cannot. Once the amino acids reach the brain, they can be converted into their respective neurotransmitters.

Although further research needs to be done, it seems that precursor therapy may be a safe and effective alternative to drugs in some cases—and in certain cases it may be even more beneficial than drug therapy.

The second orthomolecular strategy for raising brain amine levels might be called cofactor (or coenzyme) therapy. A cofactor is a compound (often a vitamin) that permits an enzyme to perform its normal biochemical functions. Without their respective cofactors, most enzymes would be inactive, and important chemical reactions would not take place. Vitamin B_6 is the cofactor for enzymes that convert tryptophan to serotonin and tyrosine to norepinephrine. A B_6 deficiency could presumably lead to depression by impairing the production of brain amines from their precursors. By the same token, vitamin B_6 supplements might favorably affect some cases of depression by raising the level of these neurotransmitters. It has been well documented that large doses of B_6 not only raise blood serotonin levels in hyperactive children, but also eliminate their symptoms in some cases (see chapter 5).

If the body's amino acids can simply be given a little "boost" with vitamin B_6, then lesser amounts of tryptophan or tyrosine might do the job, especially since the amino acids alone may not work in some cases. If there's a vitamin B_6 deficiency, a large percentage of the available tryptophan will be converted to abnormal by-products. These abnormal tryptophan metabolites may produce a paradoxical response: They may actually cause the level of serotonin in the brain to *decline*.[7] Thus, if a B_6-deficient person were to be treated with only tryptophan, then the level of brain serotonin might drop, aggravating this person's depression. On the other hand, tryptophan and B_6 together might increase the serotonin level and thereby relieve the depression.

The best therapy for some patients would probably be amino acids alone. In other cases, cofactors alone might be preferable. For still others, a combination of these molecules would be most effective. At present we do not know enough about brain biochemistry to predict the best therapy in each case. As we shall see, it's not always a good idea to use precursors and cofactors together. But if vitamin B_6 turns out to be as effective for depression as it is for certain hyperactive children, we will have another powerful and nontoxic weapon at our disposal for the treatment of this debilitating disorder.

The Evidence Behind B_6

Scientific evidence that B_6 could treat depression came from a study done in England by P. W. Adams, M.D., and co-workers.[8] They studied 22 depressed women. In each case the depression was judged to be caused by the use of birth control pills. Since oral contraceptives are known to deplete the body of vitamin B_6, Dr. Adams suspected that these episodes of depression might be due to a B_6 deficiency. Blood and urine tests determined whether the women's B_6 levels were adequate. Each woman was then given either pyridoxine hydrochloride tablets (20 milligrams twice daily) or a placebo for two months. The treatments were then reversed for an additional two months. Throughout the study neither the researchers nor the subjects were aware of the identity of the tablets.

Of the 22 women, 11 were found to have biochemical evidence of vitamin B_6 deficiency. These women experienced relief of their depression while taking B_6, but no improvement was noticed during placebo therapy. The 11 women without evidence of B_6 deficiency benefited neither from the vitamin nor from the placebo. This study demonstrated that about half of women who become depressed while taking oral contraceptives are deficient in vitamin B_6, and such patients respond to B_6 supplements.

The work of Dr. Adams's group confirmed the results of some research by Michael J. Baumblatt, M.D., and Frank Winston, M.D., in Madison, Wisconsin.[9] Fifty-eight women who were depressed and taking the Pill were treated with vitamin B_6 in doses of 25 milligrams twice daily at the first sign of any premenstrual depression. After three months of therapy, more than 75 percent of these women reported either complete relief or considerable improvement in their symptoms. The 44 women who appeared to respond to the vitamin were then asked to discontinue it for a while to see if their symptoms returned. All the women refused to do so because they were so pleased with the effects of B_6.

There was no placebo-treated control group in the study done by Drs. Baumblatt and Winston, so it's possible that some of the benefits attributed to vitamin B_6 may have actually been a placebo effect.

Still, this study is consistent with Dr. Adam's findings—strong evidence that many women suffering from contraceptive-induced depression will respond to large doses of vitamin B_6. Most depressed people are not taking birth control pills, however. Is there any evidence that they, too, are deficient in B_6 or that they might benefit from supplementation? Although the research in this area is still in its infancy, there is some indication that vitamin B_6 will eventually play a role in treating depression.

Investigators at the Virginia Polytechnic Institute and State University and at the National Institute of Mental Health (NIMH) have studied vitamin B_6 levels in depressed patients.[10] They found that plasma pyridoxal phosphate levels were about 48 percent lower in depressed patients than in controls. This difference was statistically significant. Some authorities have suggested that a plasma pyridoxal phosphate concentration of less than 8.5 nanograms per cubic centimeter (a nanogram is equivalent to one-billionth of a gram) indicates vitamin B_6 deficiency. Using this criterion, four (57 percent) of the depressed patients, but none of the controls, were deficient in B_6. The investigators also used a more sensitive method, an enzyme stimulation test, to measure vitamin B_6 levels. According to this test, all the depressed patients and none of the controls were deficient. Although only a small number of patients were studied, the evidence suggested that vitamin B_6 deficiency may be quite common in depressed individuals.

An earlier report on the B_6 levels of depressed patients was less clear-cut than the NIMH work.[11] In a 1974 study of 23 depressed patients, there was conclusive evidence of B_6 deficiency in only 1 case and suggestive evidence in another 3. The author of this study concluded that B_6 deficiency does not appear to be an important causative factor in severe cases of depression. This conclusion is open to criticism, however, because more than 1 patient out of 6 had evidence of B_6 deficiency. The possibility that vitamin B_6 might be helpful in as many as one-sixth of all cases of depression is no small matter. Some of those potential B_6 responders might be patients who either cannot tolerate or have not benefited from the usual antidepressants.

There are contradictory data on B_6 levels in women who become depressed during or just after pregnancy. In one study, deeply depressed pregnant women had significantly lower serum B_6 levels than those who were mildly depressed.[12] In another study, there was no significant difference in vitamin B_6 levels between women with postpartum (after delivery) depression and normal controls.[13] The authors of this second study concluded that "there is no evidence for vitamin B_6 deficiency in women suffering from postpartum depression." This conclusion may be partly correct. Postpartum depression seems to be caused, at least in some cases, by a deficiency of either vitamin B_{12}[14] or folate.[15] This type of depression has been relieved by correcting such deficiencies. Nevertheless, we shouldn't ignore the possibility of B_6 deficiency in women who have recently been pregnant. One of the studies mentioned above does suggest a relationship between B_6 and pregnancy depression. In addition, it's well known that some women become B_6-deficient during pregnancy.

In evaluating this research, we should remember that blood and urine measurements don't necessarily tell us what's going on in the brain. There could conceivably be a B_6 deficiency in the brain, even though blood or urine levels are normal. This localized deficiency might develop if there is a defect in the blood-brain barrier.

Certain people may be born with an abnormal enzyme in their brain that requires unusually large amounts of vitamin B_6 to function normally. If such an enzyme abnormality did exist, then depression could develop *even with normal brain levels of B_6*. In such cases, B_6 supplements would be helpful even though the patient has no actual vitamin deficiency.

Finally, vitamin B_6 deficiencies we find in depressed patients don't necessarily imply a deficiency-caused illness. One of the symptoms of depression can be loss of appetite. If someone stops eating, then nutritional deficiencies are no surprise. We cannot always be sure whether B_6 deficiency is a cause or merely a consequence of psychiatric illness.

Depression and Food Intolerance

There is recent evidence suggesting that B_6 deficiency may cause depression in at least one other group of patients. Celiac disease is a chronic illness caused by intolerance to grains containing gluten or glutenlike substances (wheat, oats, barley and rye). The most common symptoms of this disease are abdominal distention, bloating, diarrhea, weight loss and a host of other symptoms caused by malabsorption of nutrients. Celiac patients suffer massive destruction of the absorptive surface of their small bowel when they eat foods they can't tolerate. If they adhere strictly to a gluten-free diet, however, their symptoms usually disappear and their small bowel becomes normal.

Signs of mental depression are also relatively common in adults with celiac disease. One group of Swedish physicians found that the psychological features of this disease plague its victims more often than its physical symptoms. These doctors investigated the personality pattern of 11 celiac patients before and during treatment with a gluten-free diet.[16] Tested on the Minnesota Multiphasic Personality Inventory (MMPI), these patients showed evidence of suffering from depression. Those with the worst depression tended to excrete larger amounts of fat in their stools than the others, suggesting that nutritional deficiency due to malabsorption may have caused their depression. The patients took the MMPI again after staying on a gluten-free diet for one full year.

Although their physical condition had improved during this time, their depression persisted. Another group of 9 celiac patients also failed to show improvements in mood, even after five years on a gluten-free diet. Clearly, diet therapy alone failed to relieve psychological symptoms of celiac disease.

The 11 patients were then advised to take 80 milligrams of pyridoxine daily for a period of six months before taking the MMPI a third time. After six months of B_6 therapy, these patients no longer showed any evidence of depression. This study demonstrated that the depression that occurs frequently in celiac disease can be effectively treated with vitamin B_6 supplements.

Exactly why B_6 should help these patients is not clear. They were probably deficient in this vitamin from years of malabsorption. Even though the gluten-free diet improved their ability to absorb nutrients, they may have still needed supplements for a while to "catch up." It's also possible that the gluten-free diet improved intestinal function in general, but not B_6 absorption in particular. Whether these patients will continue to require B_6 therapy for relief of depression can be determined only by further research.

This study may have important implications for people other than classic celiac patients. A new concept of celiac disease has been emerging during the past decade. We now know that mild gluten intolerance exists in a relatively large segment of the population. Many people who do not have a full-blown case of celiac disease still have problems with grains containing gluten or glutenlike proteins. I have frequently seen patients with a wide range of different complaints that turned out to be caused entirely or in part by wheat or other sources of gluten. Elimination of the offending foods has completely or partly relieved symptoms in patients with recurrent canker sores, degenerative arthritis, irritable-bowel syndrome, frequent urination, hyperactivity, asthma and other problems. Although there are other causes of these symptoms, gluten intolerance is involved so often that a trial elimination diet is usually worth considering. These observations have been reported in the medical literature and have been confirmed by many practitioners of nutritional medicine. It appears that gluten intolerance is much more common than doctors had previously thought.

As we have seen, gluten intolerance is associated with both depression and vitamin B_6 deficiency. It's possible that many depressed individuals have a mild form of gluten intolerance that could lead to a mild case of vitamin B_6 deficiency. If so, B_6 therapy may be worthwhile in a relatively large number of cases.

The irritable-bowel syndrome resembles celiac disease because it is frequently associated with gluten intolerance. Irritable-bowel syndrome, also known as spastic colon or colitis, is characterized by alternating constipation and diarrhea and abdominal pain or cramping. Although most doctors believe that emotional factors are the main cause of the bowel symptoms, a recent study has shown that this is not so. In approximately two-thirds of cases studied, specific food intolerances were found to cause the symptoms. Of 21 patients tested, none of whom had celiac disease, 9 were found to react to wheat. This disorder is associated with both psychiatric symptoms and a mild form of gluten intolerance. Are some people with irritable-bowel syndrome also deficient in vitamin B_6? Will treatment with this vitamin relieve their emotional problems? These possibilities are exciting to consider, especially because irritable-bowel syndrome is so common.

Other Conditions Related to Depression

B_6 may also benefit patients with chronic renal (kidney) failure and cancer. Depression is a common feature of both of these illnesses. Vitamin B_6 deficiency frequently accompanies these diseases, too. The depression that affects victims of renal failure and cancer may be in part a reaction to the severity of their illnesses. It is also possible that correction of vitamin B_6 deficiency might relieve their depression to some extent.

Women taking estrogens to relieve menopausal symptoms and people taking isoniazid, hydralazine or penicillamine may also develop B_6 deficiency. Cigarette smokers may be low in B_6,[17] possibly because of the hydrazine compounds present in tobacco. Indeed, anyone living among the multitude of B_6 antagonists in our environment might be at risk of becoming deficient in this vitamin. Perhaps the proliferation of these antagonists in our environment is one reason the incidence of depression is increasing.

What percentage of depressed patients can expect to benefit from B_6 therapy? At present, there is no accurate way of predicting who will respond to B_6 and who will not. But certainly there are many different biochemical causes of depression—some of which could be corrected with high doses of B_6.

A Cautionary Note

An important note of caution should be injected into this discussion of vitamin B_6 and depression. For some unknown reason, an occasional depressed patient becomes definitely worse after starting vitamin B_6 therapy. At first glance it seems difficult to understand how this could happen. If B_6 raises the level of amines, and if these amines relieve depression, then B_6 should not cause a deterioration of symptoms. Yet this reaction does occur at times. There are at least two possible explanations for this paradox. One is that some cases of depression are due to an *imbalance* of brain amines, rather than a simple deficiency. Depending on an individual's biochemical makeup, B_6 therapy might increase the level of one amine more than it increases other amines. If this occurs, then the vitamin might worsen the imbalance and the depression that goes with it. Another explanation is that some people have inherited an enzyme that is especially sensitive to B_6. This enzyme might become overactive when extra B_6 is supplied. If this enzyme is present outside the brain, then it might convert most of the tryptophan and tyrosine to compounds that cannot be transported across the blood-brain barrier. Although tryptophan and tyrosine can travel easily into the brain, some of their breakdown products cannot.

These explanations are purely speculative. We obviously have quite a bit to learn about vitamin B_6, neurotransmitters and depression. As we learn more about brain biochemistry, vitamin B_6 will doubtless find a place in the management of some cases of depression. At present even the most well-informed nutritional therapists must use a great deal of guesswork. Measurement of blood serotonin levels may turn out to be useful, but there are still no clear guidelines about when to try vitamin B_6. Since this vitamin occasionally worsens the symptoms of depression, *it is unwise for the layman to experiment with B_6 without medical supervision.* Vitamin B_6 should be tried only under the watchful eye of a physician who understands the principles of orthomolecular psychiatry. It's important to note that some of the patients who are made worse by vitamin B_6 may improve when they take a combination of niacinamide and tryptophan.[18]

Although vitamin B_6 will not revolutionize the therapy of depression as the tricyclic antidepressants did, it may be beneficial in selected cases. B_6 therapy may also allow some patients to get by without the need for potentially toxic drugs. Certainly the time has come to put more research funds into the study of nontoxic therapies.

Chapter
Hyperactivity 5

It is the most common behavioral disorder of childhood, affecting an estimated 5 to 20 percent of children in the United States. It has been given at least half a dozen different names, a reflection of how little we really know about its cause. This common disorder is often a source of intense frustration for those affected and for their families, friends and teachers. For millions of American children, it causes problems in every aspect of their lives, often leading not only to poor performance in school but also to low self-esteem, unhappy personal relationships, emotional instability and uncertainty about the future.

The problem? Officially, it's called "attention deficit disorder" (ADD); yet it's also commonly known as hyperactivity, minimal brain dysfunction, hyperkinesis, minimal brain damage and brain damage behavior syndrome—terms psychiatrists now consider inappropriate. Fewer than half of all children with ADD are hyperactive, and only about 5 percent have any evidence of brain damage. The term attention deficit disorder was chosen because all affected children have one problem in common: short attention span.

Attention deficit disorder is not really a disease, with a single cause and a single cure. It is really a *syndrome*, a group of symptoms and behavior patterns that are usually found together. The most common characteristics of this syndrome are learning disabilities, short attention span, easy distractability, impulsive behavior, hyperactivity and lack of coordination.

The learning disabilities that occur with this syndrome take several forms.[1,2] Some children have difficulty receiving messages in their brain from one or more of their five senses. These problems are called perceptual disabilities. A child with a visual perceptual disability may see the letters or numbers on a printed page in reverse. *Lame* might be read as *male*, for example, or the letter *d* might appear to be a *b*. In some children this impairment in visual perception causes dyslexia (reading problems). Other children have an auditory perceptual disability (a hearing disorder), which makes it difficult for them to distinguish subtle differences in sounds. These children may misunderstand what is being said and respond inappropriately. Still others are unable to process sounds fast enough to follow ordinary conversation, so they miss part of what is being said. Another learning problem associated with ADD is known as sequencing disability; children with this problem tend to confuse which events come first when they tell a story. They may also have trouble naming the days of the week in correct order.

But the most common problem of ADD children is that they're easily distracted and have a short attention span. They have trouble finishing what they start and are hard pressed to concentrate on schoolwork or play. They also tend to be impulsive. They act before thinking, and don't seem to care if they hurt or inconvenience anyone. Emotional outbursts and temper tantrums are common, and some children fail to respond to discipline. Other symptoms and behavior patterns include stubbornness, negative attitudes, bullying, bossiness and a tendency to become frustrated easily. In addition, between 25 and 40 percent of these children are hyperactive. They have difficulty sitting still and seem to fidget constantly, run around or climb on things. Mothers complain that their child is always "into things" or is "driven by a motor."

The frustrated teacher or parent may pass off children with attention deficits as stupid or retarded. Most of the time this assessment is far from the truth. In the vast majority of cases, there is no evidence of mental retardation. In fact, some children have become totally normal once a doctor determined the cause of their disorder and provided proper treatment. It is important that the family, teachers and friends of children with ADD understand that these youngsters aren't brain-damaged or defective. Incorrectly labeling a child as hopeless will damage his self-image, blunt his ambition—and make it less likely he'll receive the medical treatment he needs. It's also unfair to label these children as "bad kids." Most of them do care and try their best to pay attention. They'd like nothing better than to succeed in their endeavors.

The reason they're inattentive isn't that they *want* to cause trouble—they simply can't keep their mind on one thing for a long period of time. Added to their concentration problems is the anxiety they feel when they're called upon to perform. These children experience many failures and have difficulty coping with most aspects of their lives. They don't deserve ridicule or disdain. What they need is compassion, understanding and patience.

What can be done to help the child with ADD? In some cases, treatment with large doses of vitamin B_6 provides great benefit. We'll discuss the use of B_6 in more detail later on. First, let's review briefly some of the other remedies, both traditional and controversial.

Psychotherapy is often recommended for the child *and* the family. The psychotherapist may be able to help everyone concerned cope better with their frustrations. In addition, special educational programs may help the child progress within the limits of his abilities.

Kindergartners on Drugs

When psychotherapy and special education aren't enough, doctors may prescribe stimulant drugs such as methylphenidate hydrochloride (Ritalin) or dextroamphetamine sulfate (Dexedrine). For some reason, stimulants slow hyperactive children down instead of speeding them up. In addition to improving behavior, these drugs also improve the child's ability to learn. Stimulants work in about 75 percent of cases of ADD. Unfortunately, they can also produce a number of disturbing side effects. Ritalin has caused loss of appetite, abdominal pain, weight loss, insomnia, increased heart rate, dizziness, headache, drowsiness, nausea, blood pressure changes and abnormal heart rhythms.[3] Dexedrine can cause as many, if not more, side effects. There have also been reports that chronic use of stimulants stunt a child's growth. Although these reports aren't conclusive, scientists haven't ruled out the possibility of growth retardation. So, despite their effectiveness, it's worrisome to see a child taking these drugs. They are among the most powerful stimulants known. Some of them are sold on the street as "speed." In fact, they're so potent and addictive that the government's Food and Drug Administration has very strict rules on when doctors may prescribe them.

Most physicians who prescribe Ritalin and other stimulants feel that their dangers have been exaggerated. They're convinced that the potential benefits outweigh the risks in children with attention disorders.

This opinion might be correct if drugs were the *only* treatment available; however, a small but growing number of physicians are convinced that dietary changes and nutritional supplements offer a promising and much safer alternative to drug therapy. In the opinion of these doctors—myself included—nutritional deficiencies, sensitivity to sugar or food additives and allergy to specific foods are involved in a large percentage of cases. Some doctors are achieving dramatic results by eliminating offending foods from the child's diet or by prescribing nutritional supplements. Unfortunately, most physicians remain resistant to the nutritional approach. They continue to prescribe dangerous drugs without even considering that a safer approach might work just as well.

Dietary Therapy

It would take a separate book to discuss in detail the scientific debate on nutrition and attention deficit disorder, but a brief account of the controversy is a must because it affects so many American families. The first suggestion that diet is related to hyperactivity came from the late Ben F. Feingold, M.D. In his 1975 book *Why Your Child Is Hyperactive*,[4] Dr. Feingold reported that a class of chemicals called salicylates caused hyperactivity in some children. A number of widely used food colorings contain a salicylate molecule. These chemicals also occur naturally in certain foods, such as oranges, apples, grapes and almonds. Dr. Feingold found that the behavior of some children improved dramatically when they eliminated all salicylate-containing foods from their diet. Feingold's work received a great deal of publicity. Parents began to experiment with the salicylate-free diet, and many discovered that it worked. Before long, "Feingold Associations" were forming all around the country, as parents tried to spread the word about the benefits of the Feingold diet.

Doctors then began performing controlled studies to determine whether these alleged benefits were really due to the diet or were just a placebo effect. (Let me pause for a minute and explain two of the medical terms I used in that last sentence. In a *controlled study*, two groups are tested: One group receives the real treatment; the other group [the control group] receives a fake treatment [placebo] they think is real. If the "real" group does a lot better on the treatment than the control group, chances are the treatment really works. If they don't, chances are the changes for the better that *do* occur are caused by the *placebo effect*—it wasn't the treatment that caused the change but a *belief* in it, an expectation that it would work that produced the results.) To date, a dozen or more studies have been done. The consensus from this research is that food colorings are important in only a small minority of children.[5] Under controlled conditions, these additives usually didn't aggravate hyperactivity. Because carefully controlled studies couldn't confirm the dramatic results reported by Dr. Feingold, most pediatricians became disillusioned with the whole idea that diet is an important factor.

But any physician who has made a serious effort at testing the nutritional approach on his patients knows that it's frequently very helpful. The fact that food colorings aren't usually involved doesn't rule out the importance of other dietary components. Dr. Feingold was on the right track when he claimed that salicylates aggravate hyperactivity, but he isolated only a small part of the problem. Nutrition-oriented doctors are convinced that sensitivity to *refined sugar* is an important factor in a large percentage of cases. The behavioral problems of some children can be controlled as long as they stay away from all refined sugar. But as soon as they eat a candy bar or drink a soft drink, their symptoms return in full force. At present, there's only one published study concerning the effect of sugar on hyperactive children. Ronald Prinz, Ph.D., and co-workers at the University of South Carolina found that hyperactive children eat diets containing far more sugar than do normal children.[6] Yet even though there hasn't been much scientific research on the subject, the observations about sugar are no less valid. Mothers of ADD children consistently report that their normally well-behaved kids become uncontrollable every time they eat something with sugar in it. These statements are hard to ignore.

Part of the reason the Feingold diet works may be because it's low in sugar. Many foods that have coloring agents also have lots of sugar. When food colorings are removed from a child's diet, much of the sugar is removed at the same time. So Dr. Feingold's observations were valid, even though the explanation for his findings was only partly correct.

In other children, allergy to specific foods seems to be an important cause of inattentiveness.[7] Common foods such as dairy products, wheat, citrus fruits, corn and eggs may trigger symptoms in children sensitive to them. When these foods are eliminated from the child's diet, symptoms improve or disappear.

I want to emphasize that it's extremely difficult to prove scientifically the importance of diet. Dietary treatment is usually individualized and is sometimes complicated. That makes it virtually impossible to satisfy the demand of modern science that half the children in a study of ADD be treated with an *identical* placebo, a substance that looks and tastes like the real treatment. How do you make oatmeal taste like chocolate bars?

Even though firm scientific proof is lacking, it's the honest belief of hundreds of doctors that nutritional therapy works. Skeptical physicians have nothing to lose by experimenting with this nontoxic treatment. Those willing to try something new will almost certainly find that many of their patients improve. They will also need to prescribe dangerous drugs far less often.

It's exciting to see the improvements that occur when a child eliminates sugar, allergenic foods and additives from his diet. Nothing, however, works all the time. Some children continue to do poorly even with appropriate diet and drug therapy. That's where vitamin B_6 comes in. Supplements of the nutrient work in some cases where nothing else helps. And even for some children who have responded to stimulants, vitamin B_6 may be a safer and more effective alternative.

B_6 and Hyperactivity

The possibility that vitamin B_6 might be related to hyperactivity occurred to Mary Coleman, M.D., about a decade ago. Along with her colleague Alan S. Greenberg, M.D., Dr. Coleman had been measuring blood serotonin levels in a group of mentally retarded institutionalized patients. Serotonin, as I explained in chapter 4, is a molecule normally present in the brain that is believed to play a role in various psychological disorders. Out of 30 patients Dr. Coleman studied, all of whom were severly hyperactive and emotionally disturbed, 83 percent had serotonin levels below normal.[8]

These patients were treated with various antipsychotic drugs in an attempt to improve their symptoms. The only drugs that worked were those that also raised the serotonin level. Medications that didn't increase blood serotonin didn't relieve symptoms. Dr. Coleman later found that blood serotonin levels were also depressed in hyperactive children. As many as 88 percent of such children had levels below normal.[9]

The work of Dr. Coleman and her co-workers showed that serotonin might play a key role in many cases of ADD. And if low serotonin is the cause of symptoms in these children, then vitamin B_6 might relieve the symptoms by raising serotonin levels. As I noted in chapters 2 and 4, vitamin B_6 has an important effect on serotonin metabolism. One, it activates the enzymes that are responsible for converting the amino acid tryptophan into serotonin.[10] If insufficient amounts of this vitamin are present, then serotonin production will be impaired. Two, tryptophan may be converted into many different metabolites (by-products), and the amount of B_6 present determines the extent to which some of these metabolites are produced. B_6-deficient people excrete (and presumably manufacture) unusually large amounts of xanthurenic acid, kynurenine and 3-hydroxykynurenine. People with normal B_6 levels, on the other hand, excrete normal amounts of these metabolites.[11] It seems that two of these tryptophan metabolites (kynurenine and 3-hydroxykynurenine) somehow cause the level of serotonin in the brain to decline.[12] In short, vitamin B_6 activates the enzymes necessary to synthesize serotonin and also prevents the production of those tryptophan by-products that interfere with serotonin.

Dr. Coleman and her colleagues found that large doses of B_6 do indeed raise blood serotonin levels.[13] The increase occurred whether the levels were initially low, normal or elevated. It appeared that B_6 supplements might relieve the symptoms of hyperactive children.

But that study was only the first step. To determine whether B_6 *really* worked, Dr. Coleman recruited six children with moderate or severe hyperactivity.[13] All of them had normal intelligence *and* low blood levels of serotonin. In addition, each of them had been treated with Ritalin and had improved while on this medication. They ranged in age from 8 to 13.

The 21-week study was divided into seven 3-week periods. The children received a different medication during each of these periods. For half the children, the sequence of medications was: placebo, low-dose pyridoxine, high-dose pyridoxine, placebo, low-dose Ritalin, high-dose Ritalin and placebo. For the rest of the children, the treatment sequence was similar, except they received Ritalin before B_6. The dosages of B_6 were chosen individually for each patient and were based on a combination of clinical history and blood serotonin level. One dose (10 to 15 milligrams of B_6 per kilogram of body weight a day, about 425 milligrams for a 75-pound child) was designed to be less than optimal. The other dose (15 to 30 milligrams per kilogram a day, about 750 milligrams for a 75-pound child) was presumed to be the optimal dosage. (This is a large amount, and should be taken *only* under a doctor's supervision.) The amount of Ritalin prescribed was also based on clinical history. As with B_6, one dosage of Ritalin was suboptimal and the other was optimal. The value of each treatment was assessed by a behavior rating scale. Items on the scale included restlessness, excitability, short attention span, tendency to become frustrated, drastic mood changes and temper outbursts.

When the results were tabulated, it turned out that the best behavior was evident during treatment with high doses of B_6. Smaller amounts of B_6, on the other hand, weren't any more effective than the placebo. The second-best behavior ratings occurred when Ritalin was given. The children did worst during the placebo periods. The conclusion? High doses of B_6 were judged to be slightly more effective than Ritalin, *even though each child had previously responded to the stimulant drug*. In addition, B_6 supplements raised blood serotonin levels; Ritalin did not. Apparently, Ritalin affects hyperactivity in some way that's unrelated to serotonin metabolism. The effect of B_6 lasted for about three weeks after the vitamin was discontinued.

The results of this study suggest that vitamin B_6 therapy may be of great value for hyperactive children who have low serotonin levels. Dr. Coleman's work introduced an exciting new approach to the treatment of attention deficit disorder. Vitamin B_6 appears to be safer than Ritalin. So in cases where these two substances are equally effective, B_6 would be preferable to the stimulant.

There was one problem with Dr. Coleman's study. An analysis of the data showed that there was a 10 percent probability ($p = .10$) that the benefits attributed to B_6 were actually due to chance. In the language of science, the results were not "statistically significant." In other words, we can be only 90 percent certain that the effect of B_6 was real. Scientists like to be 95 percent ($p = .05$) sure before they agree that a treatment is effective. According to the rigid rules of modern science, Dr. Coleman's data didn't prove that vitamin B_6 works.

Despite this seeming lack of firm proof, the potential of B_6 shouldn't be ignored. This vitamin could work in selected cases, and it is apparently safer than the drugs now used for hyperactive children. A safe and *possibly* effective treatment is often preferable to a dangerous drug of *proven* value. Unfortunately, most doctors don't believe that B_6 is even possibly effective.

There are two main reasons that B_6 hasn't been given the attention it deserves. First, most doctors are unaware of the research suggesting it may be helpful. Physicians usually read no more than a few medical journals every week. Since Dr. Coleman's study was published in a somewhat obscure journal, *Biological Psychiatry*, it's gone unnoticed for the most part. The only exposure most physicians have had to vitamin therapy is through review articles in traditional journals, and these articles rarely do justice to the subject. For example, a 1979 review of attention deficit disorder offered the following analysis: "The use of megavitamins, trace elements, or the elimination of specific food additives has been proposed as a treatment for hyperactivity. These approaches have not been successful."[2] When uncritical and biased statements like this one are all most doctors have to go on, it's no wonder they shun vitamin therapy.

The second reason B_6 has been ignored (assuming that some physicians have read Dr. Coleman's report) is that many doctors don't understand statistics. There is a common misconception in medicine concerning the meaning of "statistical significance." Most physicians have the mistaken impression that failure to show statistical significance is the same as proving the treatment didn't work. In other words, if you are less than 95 percent sure that B_6 was effective, then you must conclude it was *ineffective*. Although this reasoning is incorrect, doctors have made this same mistake time after time. They forget that statistical significance has as much to do with the number of subjects studied as it does with the value of the therapy. When a small number of patients are involved, even a dramatic effect may not achieve statistical significance.

A 1981 article published in the *Archives of Internal Medicine* pointed out just how often we toss potentially beneficial remedies onto the junk heap. Three hundred thirty-five published articles that contained "negative" results were reexamined. It was found that, because of inadequate sample size, a small beneficial effect would have been missed 86 percent of the time. Even major clinical improvements would have been missed 38 percent of the time if the sole criterion for success were statistical significance.[14]

The purpose of making all this fuss about statistical significance is to point out that Dr. Coleman's work should be taken seriously. Based on her data, the following statements can be made: (1) vitamin B_6 was far superior to a placebo; (2) there is a nine out of ten probability that the effect of B_6 was not due to chance; and (3) B_6 worked at least as well as, and possibly better than, Ritalin. When put this way, B_6 appears to have great potential.

No doctor should be faulted for experimenting with vitamin B_6 or other nontoxic therapies when the only alternative is Ritalin or another dangerous stimulant. As long as the doctor and the patient's family are honest in their evaluation, the results should speak for themselves.

There is no doubt that hard-nosed skeptics will continue to reject the use of B_6 until a large-scale study proves its effectiveness. Without begrudging them their skepticism, I want to remind them of the first rule of medicine: "Above all, do no harm." Stimulants can always be prescribed later, if diet and vitamin therapy have not helped.

A Pediatrician Who Prescribes B_6

One physician who has looked seriously at B_6 is Arnold Brenner, M.D., a pediatrician from Randallstown, Maryland. Dr. Brenner's interest in this vitamin was stimulated by a chance observation in 1971.[15] A three-year-old girl with a history of irritability, hostile outbursts and temper tantrums was hospitalized because of persistent abdominal pain. During the course of her evaluation, she was found to have a positive tuberculin skin test, indicating she had been exposed to tuberculosis. The girl was therefore given isoniazid (INH), an antituberculous medication. Within a week she developed insomnia and her behavior became much worse. Because INH is known to interfere with vitamin B_6, Dr. Brenner suspected that a B_6 deficiency might be at the root of her behavioral changes. He found that 100 milligrams of B_6 a day reduced the child's irritability. But he had to increase the daily dose to 400 milligrams before her symptoms were controlled completely. (These amounts should be taken only under a doctor's supervision.) After six months, both INH and B_6 were discontinued. Three weeks later, the abnormal behavior returned. The child's mother described her daughter as "wild, easily distracted and disruptive." Vitamin B_6 in daily doses of 200 to 400 milligrams again controlled her behavior. Over the next 13 years,[16] the child has required continuous treatment with B_6. As long as she takes the vitamin (currently 200 milligrams a day), her behavior remains normal. When she stops or when a placebo is given instead of B_6, she becomes irritable, hostile, hyperactive and aggressive.

Dr. Brenner tried giving large doses of B_6 to several other patients with similar symptoms. In some of these cases, there was a dramatic disappearance of hyperactivity. In others, there was no effect. Interestingly, B_6 appeared to make some children markedly worse. One of the children made worse by B_6 was then given thiamine (vitamin B_1), which completely controlled all behavioral problems.

Around the same time Dr. Brenner was discovering the value of vitamin therapy, other doctors were beginning to report that high doses of niacinamide and other vitamins benefited children with learning disabilities. So Dr. Brenner decided to study the effect of individual vitamins on 100 of his patients with attention deficit disorder.[17] Each was given a separate three-day trial with large doses of thiamine, pantothenic acid, pyridoxine and placebo. If a specific vitamin brought about a dramatic improvement, its use was continued. If no response was noted, then niacinamide, combinations of B vitamins or elimination diets were tried.

Of the 100 children tested, 9 responded dramatically to vitamin B_6 (at a dose of 300 milligrams a day). An additional 5 responded only after receiving larger doses of B_6, ranging from 500 to 2,000 milligrams a day. (Once again, these large dosages—while effective—must be taken only while under a doctor's care.) Some of these 14 patients also required additional vitamins and minerals to obtain maximal benefit. Eight other children responded dramatically to thiamine, and 11 improved after taking either niacinamide or a combination of B vitamins and minerals. Eight children improved after dietary changes alone.

Dr. Brenner also observed several interesting nutrient interactions. Half the children who had improved with thiamine therapy worsened when they were given B_6. Conversely, half the B_6 responders worsened during thiamine treatment. Most of those who had improved with B_6 eventually relapsed without warning and for no apparent reason. It was later discovered that blood levels of zinc had fallen during B_6 therapy. When a zinc supplement was added to the B_6, symptoms again disappeared.

The study done by Dr. Brenner provided some important information. Attention deficit disorder appears to have many different causes. A significant number of cases respond to large amounts of one or more vitamins. B_6 was most often effective, but some children benefited only from thiamine, niacinamide or a combination of nutrients. Notably, certain vitamins made some children worse. In general there was no way of predicting who would respond to which vitamins. But like Dr. Coleman, Dr. Brenner found that children with low serotonin levels were likely to respond to B_6. Conversely, those with elevated blood serotonin sometimes became worse when they were given B_6.

It seems worthwhile to measure blood serotonin in children with attention deficit disorder. If the value is low, then B_6 should be tried. If serotonin is normal or high, then perhaps dietary treatment or some combination of vitamins and minerals might help. A blood test for serotonin costs about $100. But considering the benefits it could bring, it's likely to be worth the expense. Future studies to assess the value of B_6 should concentrate on children with low blood serotonin levels.

I'd like to make a few other comments about vitamin treatment of hyperactive children. It's likely that some children will respond to diet *and* vitamins. The vitamins may work in some cases by blocking an adverse reaction to offending foods or additives. For example, vitamin B_6 might prevent symptoms caused by the ingestion of tartrazine (FD&C Yellow No. 5). This frequently used food additive is converted by the body into a hydrazine molecule,[18] which almost certainly interferes with vitamin B_6 (see chapter 1). Some cases of apparent tartrazine sensitivity may actually represent tartrazine-induced B_6 deficiency. If so, then symptoms may be relieved either by taking B_6 or by eliminating food dyes from the diet.

Changing your child's diet is better than having him take B_6. While B_6 therapy *appears* to be safe within the limits described in this chapter, we still don't know if there are subtle adverse effects from long-term use. As Dr. Brenner discovered, large doses of vitamins can cause imbalances of other nutrients. And the "wrong" vitamins can make some children worse. If dietary therapy doesn't work, *then* try supplements. Some children may need both approaches to achieve best results. If B_6 or other vitamins are necessary, use the lowest effective dose. This dose will vary from person to person. Vitamin therapy can be extremely complicated. If can also be harmful if abused. So—it's very important that you consult with a nutrition-oriented physician before embarking on vitamin therapy.

I want to mention one last point. We don't know for sure whether B_6 works by raising serotonin levels or by some other mechanism. There are other molecules in the brain, such as dopamine and epinephrine, that are affected by B_6 supplements. These molecules may also play a role in psychological disorders. But the mechanics of improvement aren't really important. What *is* important is that B_6 produces dramatic benefits for as many as one out of seven children with ADD.

Chapter

Other Emotional Disorders 6

Autism

The term *autism,* which means "preoccupation with the self," refers to a severe psychiatric disorder, usually of childhood. Autistic children withdraw from contact with people, including their parents, and tend to develop affectionate relationships with inanimate objects. They either fail to speak at all or develop an incomprehensible private language. In some cases, autistic children rock incessantly back and forth, and drool, grunt or mutter animallike sounds. Autistic children may scratch, bite or slap themselves, even drawing blood without apparent pain. Although they may seem aware of other people, they make no attempt to relate to them. Autism is obviously a serious problem for both the children and their families.

The cause of autism is unknown. Some evidence suggests that abnormal physical development is at fault, while other studies implicate severe emotional trauma in infancy. In many autistic children, the cause seems to be a combination of physical and emotional factors.

It's conceivable that any number of biochemical abnormalities in the brain could lead to autistic behavior. Some research suggests that vitamin B_6 deficiency or dependency may be one such factor.

In 1966 British doctors studied tryptophan metabolism in a group of 16 psychotic children (including autistic children).[1] After they took tryptophan, 9 of these children excreted abnormal metabolites (break-

down products), suggesting that their bodies were low in B$_6$. When 4
of the 9 children took vitamin B$_6$ supplements, their tryptophan metabolism became normal. More than half the children were either deficient in B$_6$ or needed unusually large amounts of this vitamin. Abnormal
vitamin B$_6$ metabolism tended to occur most often in children whose
problems began in their earliest years.

Vitamin B$_6$ influences the brain's biochemistry in many ways, including its production of serotonin and dopamine. Because the levels
of these chemical messengers are reportedly low in some autistic children,[2] B$_6$ supplements might be helpful in some cases. Bernard Rimland,
Ph.D., of the Institute for Child Behavior Research in San Diego, became interested in vitamin therapy after receiving numerous letters from
parents who were excited over how vitamins had helped their children.
To follow up these interesting observations, Dr. Rimland tested the
effect of various B vitamins and vitamin C on psychotic children, including 191 autistic children. He was impressed by the frequency with
which vitamin therapy appeared to improve both behavior and physical
well-being in these children.[3] Dr. Rimland and several colleagues decided to solidify their impressions with a carefully controlled double-
blind study.[2] They studied 16 autistic children who had improved on
B$_6$ administered in dosages ranging from 75 to 3,000 milligrams a day.
All were taking other vitamins and minerals, and some were also taking
drugs. Each child continued to receive the usual dose of B$_6$ during one
part of the study, but took a placebo during another part. According to
behavior ratings by parents and teachers, the children's behavior deteriorated significantly when B$_6$ was replaced by the placebo. This study
confirmed Dr. Rimland's initial observation that vitamin B$_6$ improves
the behavior of some autistic children.

More recently, vitamin B$_6$ supplements were given to 44 autistic
children in France[4] who took daily 30-milligram doses of B$_6$ for each
kilogram of body weight. Dr. Rimland had found earlier that B$_6$ in high
doses would occasionally make children wet their beds and become more
irritable and sound-sensitive. These side effects could be prevented by
adding a magnesium supplement, so the French researchers included
magnesium lactate (400 or 500 milligrams a day). Of 44 children, 15
improved while taking B$_6$ and magnesium. They became more alert,
had fewer emotional outbursts and were less likely to mutilate themselves. When the supplements were discontinued at the end of the
study, their behavior deteriorated. The children who had responded to
B$_6$ were retested in a double-blind trial, which confirmed the impressions from the earlier trial.

Apparently, vitamin B₆ supplements, along with magnesium, help about one-third of autistic children. The scientists who have studied B₆ emphasize that it's not a cure for autism but may improve behavior in certain cases. Magnesium supplements might conceivably enhance the effects of B₆, since these two nutrients work together in so many ways. Because large doses of B₆ are needed to treat the autistic child, such therapy should not be attempted without the advice of a physician.

Breath-Holding Spells

Physical or emotional pain commonly triggers breath-holding spells in some children. Although this condition apparently doesn't produce serious harm, it's alarming for parents to see their child turn slightly blue or even pass out. Various treatments have been tried for children who hold their breath, but none have been effective. M. K. Abecasis, M.D., a Portuguese pediatrician, has found that vitamin B₆ supplements eliminate breath-holding spells in some children.[5] After ten years of experience with B₆ therapy, Dr. Abecasis reported that the results were "very satisfactory." The doctor used 40-milligram dosages once a day for children up to the age of two, and twice a day for older children. Treatment was usually continued for a month. One child studied in the laboratory had an abnormal tryptophan load test suggestive of B₆ deficiency. After treatment with the vitamin, the child's breath-holding spells diminished rapidly and his tryptophan load test became normal.

Schizophrenia

Schizophrenia is perhaps the most devastating of all mental illnesses. Victims of chronic schizophrenia occupy more than half of all the beds in psychiatric hospitals around the country. Although the discovery of major tranquilizers (chlorpromazine, haloperidol, thiothixene, etc.) was a major advance in the treatment of schizophrenia, many who suffer from this illness remain confined to institutions or are barely able to cope in the outside world. Schizophrenics tend to withdraw from other people into a world of unrealistic fantasies and delusions. They don't withdraw deliberately; rather, they seem to have no control over their actions. In some forms of schizophrenia, the patients' emotions become dulled and their faces take on a rigid expression. Their emotional responses may seem wildly inappropriate—laughter at the news of someone's death or anger for no apparent reason. Locked inside their own world, schizophrenics are frequently a burden to themselves, their family and society.

Psychiatrists used to assume that schizophrenia was caused by traumatic emotional events from early childhood. It now appears, however, that biochemical rather than purely psychological factors are a major part of this serious mental illness. Apparently, the thought patterns typical of schizophrenia result from the presence of abnormal molecules in the brain. Of course, anyone whose brain chemistry causes him to think and behave the way a schizophrenic does is bound to develop secondary psychological problems. It appears, though, that the best chance of solving the riddle of schizophrenia is to identify and correct the biochemical factors that cause abnormal thinking. The powerful "antipsychotic" drugs used to treat schizophrenics act by altering the metabolism of certain chemical messengers in the brain.

Since certain vitamins and minerals also influence brain biochemistry, some doctors and scientists have attempted to treat schizophrenia nutritionally. Several decades ago, Abram Hoffer, Ph.D., M.D., and Humphrey Osmond, M.D., found that large doses of niacinamide were helpful in some cases. Vitamin C also appeared to increase the effectiveness of niacinamide in many instances. Little attention was initially given to the work of Drs. Hoffer and Osmond; however, interest in vitamin treatment of mental illness increased after two-time Nobel laureate Linus Pauling, Ph.D., published a landmark article on the subject in 1968. Writing in the respected journal *Science*, Dr. Pauling introduced the concept of "orthomolecular psychiatric therapy,"[6] and argued that mental illness might be effectively treated by adjusting the concentration of molecules normally present in the human body.

Carl Pfeiffer, M.D., Ph.D., director of the Brain Bio Center in Princeton, New Jersey, took the concept of orthomolecular psychiatry a step further.[7] Dr. Pfeiffer believed that any number of abnormalities of brain biochemistry could cause the symptoms and behavior patterns that we call schizophrenia. After carefully studying a number of outpatient schizophrenics, Dr. Pfeiffer and colleagues used laboratory tests to identify certain abnormalities that allowed them to divide their patients into three categories. One group had an abnormally low level of a compound called histamine in their blood, while a second group had an unusually high amount of this chemical. When these patients were given treatment designed to bring their blood histamine level back to normal, most of them improved.

A third group of schizophrenics (about 35 percent of the patients) had normal blood histamine levels but were excreting an abnormal chemical in their urine called kryptopyrrole (KP). Exactly why some schizophrenics were "pyroluric" (excreting KP in their urine) was unclear.

However, Dr. Pfeiffer discovered that KP forms a chemical bond with vitamin B_6 and zinc, and carries these important nutrients out of the body with it. Vitamin B_6 and zinc are both known to influence key metabolic reactions in the brain. Perhaps, Dr. Pfeiffer thought, KP was provoking schizophrenic symptoms by causing a deficiency of these nutrients. Dr. Pfeiffer began giving B_6 and zinc supplements to those of his schizophrenic patients who were excreting KP. The results were exciting. After treating more than 300 pyroluric patients, Dr. Pfeiffer confidently wrote: "The B_6 and zinc treatment is usually effective in producing a remission of their psychosis." Symptoms would return whenever the patient discontinued or ran out of the supplements.[7]

The discovery that more than 30 percent of schizophrenics would respond to a simple nutritional regimen was a major advance. The successful use of B_6 and zinc where antipsychotic drugs and electric shock had previously failed should have generated widespread enthusiasm among the orthodox psychiatric community. Instead, this treatment and others currently used by the small group known as orthomolecular psychiatrists have been the subject of bitter controversy for more than a decade. Several Canadian physicians reported only minor improvements in schizophrenics treated with B_6, far less improvement than Dr. Pfeiffer had found.[8] There were probably two reasons for the discrepancy. First, the Canadian group did not limit their study to pyroluric patients, so their results were diluted by a large number of patients who could not be expected to respond to Dr. Pfeiffer's treatment. Second, the Canadian group used only 75 milligrams of B_6 a day and no zinc, while Dr. Pfeiffer found that larger doses of B_6 were often needed (sometimes as much as 3,000 milligrams a day) to produce good results. He also prescribed additional supplements to some patients.

Dr. Pfeiffer was convinced that the way KP caused symptoms was by pulling B_6 and zinc out of the body through the urine. However, the amount of B_6 that KP took with it was usually no more than a few milligrams a day. If Dr. Pfeiffer's explanation were correct, it would be hard to understand how several thousand or even several hundred milligrams of this vitamin could be needed to produce improvements.

There is another, more likely explanation for KP's toxic effects: Compounds that chemically link up with B_6 are sometimes capable of interfering with the metabolism of this vitamin. You may recall that pyridoxyl-lysine, formed during food processing, is a B_6 antimetabolite. Perhaps B_6-KP-zinc molecules also interfere with the functions of B_6. If these molecules inhibit one or more B_6-dependent enzymes, then (as we saw in chapter 1) a very large dose of B_6 might be required to counteract their effects. When other investigators decide to study B_6 and zinc therapy, it's important that they use the doses Dr. Pfeiffer found to be necessary; otherwise, the results will be unimpressive. Perhaps this alternative explanation of Dr. Pfeiffer's data will help skeptical scientists accept his observation that very large amounts of B_6 are needed.

While traditional psychiatrists have largely rejected Dr. Pfeiffer's work, none of them have bothered to repeat his research. Instead, they cling to their usual argument that it is the job of the orthomolecular psychiatrists to prove their claims in double-blind studies. Unfortunately, those who are challenging the orthodoxy are not in a financial position to set up large clinical trials. Even if they were, most of the "new breed," after having seen how much their treatments help, would consider it unethical to give half their patients a placebo. It seems that the controversy will not soon be resolved.

Fortunately, more doctors are becoming interested in alternative treatments of mental illness, and a few insurance companies are starting to pay for vitamin therapy. Still, there is a good deal of research that needs to be done. Orthomolecular treatment of schizophrenia has become quite complicated. Some patients are given large doses of niacinamide and ascorbic acid. Others are treated with B_6 and zinc. Still others apparently improve when they eliminate milk and wheat from their diet. More recently, some doctors have found that *Candida albicans,* a common yeast organism, can trigger schizophrenia, apparently by setting off an allergic reaction in the brain. Selected individuals have improved dramatically after taking a drug that eradicates *Candida albicans*.

Schizophrenics should *not* attempt to treat themselves with large doses of vitamins. Large doses of niacinamide, for example, can cause liver damage and other side effects if they aren't monitored carefully. Dr. Pfeiffer has pointed out that serious consequences can also result if a schizophrenic abruptly discontinues high-dose vitamin B_6 therapy. Without proper testing, neither a schizophrenic nor his family would know which of the half a dozen or so orthmolecular treatments is most likely to work. As more doctors become interested in alternative treatments of schizophrenia, an orthomolecular therapist will soon be easier to find.

Side Effects from Tranquilizers

A certain class of so-called antipsychotic drugs is used to alter the abnormal thought patterns of schizophrenics and other psychotics. These drugs, often referred to as "major tranquilizers," are also used to control nausea and vomiting and to relieve neurotic anxiety and tension. With prolonged use, any of the major tranquilizers can cause rather severe neurological side effects. One syndrome induced by these drugs is tardive dyskinesia. As many as 20 percent of chronically institutionalized patients suffer from this side effect of their medication. People with tardive dyskinesia tend to develop repetitive involuntary movements, such as sucking and smacking of the lips, jaw and tongue movements, and back-and-forth movements of the arms or legs. For many, tardive dyskinesia is irreversible, and drug treatment is only modestly successful.

Doctors have noted similarities between people with tardive dyskinesia and those who have taken an overdose of the drug L-dopa (used to treat Parkinson's disease). Because vitamin B_6 can reverse the symptoms of L-dopa intoxication, a psychiatrist from Syracuse, New York, attempted to treat tardive dyskinesia with B_6 as well.[9] Joseph DeVeaugh-Geiss, M.D., was aware that previous studies had shown that B_6 did little for this neurological syndrome. In these negative studies only 200 to 300 milligrams of pyridoxine were used each day, however.

Figuring that higher doses might work better, Dr. DeVeaugh-Geiss persuaded five patients suffering from tardive dyskinesia to take a daily dose of 1,000 to 1,400 milligrams of B_6. Four of these five patients suffered fewer involuntary movements. The improvement usually occurred within a week of starting the vitamin and was maintained as long as therapy was continued (4 to 12 weeks). When the B_6 was stopped, a relapse occurred within 1 week.

Of course, one must always be cautious when using such large amounts of B_6. Although the vitamin dosage that relieved tardive dyskinesia is below the range reported to cause B_6 toxicity (2,000 to 6,000 milligrams a day), B_6 treatment should be undertaken only under a doctor's supervision.

Some investigators have found that lecithin supplements can suppress tardive dyskinesia, although others have not found this treatment worthwhile. Perhaps a combination of lecithin and vitamin B_6 (possibly even a dose lower than 1,000 milligrams a day) will also turn out to be beneficial.

Part IV

Thwarting the Killers, Banishing Pain

Chapter

Heart 7
Disease

Cardiovascular disease remains the number one killer in the United States. Each year nearly one million Americans die from heart attacks and other cardiovascular problems, and thousands of others become incapacitated by chronic chest pain, breathing difficulties and other symptoms related to a failing cardiovascular system. Diseases of the heart and blood vessels cost an estimated $50 billion a year in medical expenses and reduced productivity.

Heart attacks are usually, though not always, associated with atherosclerosis (hardening of the arteries), a disease in which plaques, composed of cholesterol, other fats, calcium, and fibrous tissue, accumulate on the inside wall of arteries and restrict the passage of blood. If the accumulation of plaques goes unchecked, it restricts the blood flow that carries oxygen and vital nutrients to the tissues and organs. At some point, if the blood flow becomes critically low, the tissues it nourishes starve and die. That means that if a coronary artery becomes blocked, a portion of the heart muscle (myocardium) may die (myocardial infarction, or heart attack).

Risk Factors and Causes

Heart disease is a disease of modern civilization. Although it's rare in nonindustrialized countries, it becomes increasingly common as these nations adopt a more Westernized life-style. Exactly which aspects of modern living lead to cardiovascular disease has stimulated decades of research and much lively debate. No single theory can explain all we know about heart disease, and it's likely that many factors contribute to this modern epidemic.

In an attempt to understand the causes of heart disease, scientists have developed a list of risk factors. For instance, we find that people with high levels of serum cholesterol, uric acid, triglycerides or glucose are more likely to die of a heart attack than those without these laboratory abnormalities. Smokers and people with high blood pressure, diabetes or a stress-evoking personality pattern known as Type A are also at increased risk. The main thrust of the traditional approach to preventing heart disease has been to eliminate these risk factors. Lowering serum cholesterol and blood pressure and quitting smoking are frequently promoted as ways to avoid a heart attack.

A risk factor is not necessarily the same as a cause, however. Suppose, for example, that vitamin B_6 deficiency leads to heart attacks (there is evidence that it does). Suppose also that lack of vitamin B_6 causes the serum cholesterol to rise (animal studies suggest that it does).[1] People low in vitamin B_6 might have both high serum cholesterol and an increased risk of heart attack. Elevated serum cholesterol would therefore be a risk factor for heart disease, even though vitamin B_6 deficiency is really the cause. If we take steps merely to reduce the serum cholesterol without determining why it's elevated, we can't expect to solve the problem of heart disease. We must begin thinking in terms of the *causes* of heart disease, rather than looking only at risk factors.

The danger of relying on risk factors was illustrated by the results of a 1965 British study. Men suffering from heart disease were divided into two groups: half the men consumed a diet high in saturated fat and cholesterol; the other half ate a low-fat diet supplemented with about four tablespoons of corn oil a day. Corn oil is usually thought of as helpful for the heart because it lowers serum cholesterol, one of the risk factors for heart disease. During the two-year study, the men taking corn oil did in fact have lower serum cholesterol than the men eating eggs, butter, bacon and other allegedly dangerous foods; however, nearly twice as many men who consumed corn oil (48 percent) suffered a "major cardiac event" during the study as those who ate the high-animal-fat diet.[2] (On the other hand, a different study lasting ten years and involving many people *did* show a sharp reduction in heart attacks among those who substituted vegetable fats for animal fats.[3] Obviously, the last word on vegetable oils has yet to be spoken.)

The MR FIT (Multiple Risk Factor Intervention Trial) study further illustrates the limitations of risk-factor analysis. This was a $115 million study designed to answer the question, once and for all, of whether modifying risk factors will prevent heart attacks.[4] Twelve thousand middle-aged men who had at least one risk factor (high blood pressure, cholesterol, etc.) for developing a heart attack were studied. Half the men were taught how to lower their blood pressure and their serum cholesterol by consuming less salt, saturated fat and cholesterol, and more polyunsaturated fat. They were also counseled individually on the importance of quitting smoking and, when necessary, were given medication to lower their blood pressure. The other half of the men were not given any specific advice but were referred for usual medical care in the community.

The men who had been counseled achieved lower serum cholesterol and blood pressure than those who had been referred for community care. In addition, fewer of the counseled men were still smoking by the end of the study. The researchers' intervention had clearly succeeded in modifying risk factors. Still, death from cardiovascular disease was approximately the same in both groups. The results of the study were complicated by an unexpectedly high death rate in men taking diuretics (water pills) for their high blood pressure. Nevertheless, this expensive and carefully designed experiment provided little support for the notion that we can prevent heart attacks by cutting down on dietary cholesterol, saturated fat, salt and cigarettes.

The Lipid Hypothesis

The MR FIT study dealt a major blow to the so-called "lipid hypothesis": the theory that heart and blood vessel disease is caused by eating too much meat, eggs, butter, whole milk and other fatty foods. On the other hand, the MR FIT failure wasn't surprising to the minority of scientists who had argued for years that the lipid hypothesis was flawed. On the surface, this hypothesis seemed so simple and logical that it was difficult to reject, even in the face of numerous inconsistencies and unexplainable facts.

The lipid hypothesis is based on four major observations:

1. populations with high death rates from coronary artery disease consume large amounts of cholesterol and saturated fat;

2. dietary cholesterol and saturated fat raise serum cholesterol, while polyunsaturated fat lowers it;

3. atherosclerotic plaques (fatty deposits in the arteries) contain cholesterol;

4. feeding large amounts of cholesterol to animals produces fatty deposits in their arteries.

The lipid hypothesis itself states: *A diet high in cholesterol and saturated fat causes an increase in the serum cholesterol level, which in turn leads to atherosclerosis (hardening of the arteries) and its complications (heart attacks and strokes).* Although the lipid hypothesis seems to flow directly from the four observations, each observation either has serious weaknesses or can be explained without the lipid hypothesis.[5]

One international survey did show a positive correlation between national heart disease rates and animal-fat consumption, but there are many other factors, not all dietary, that are also associated with this disease. Why blame animal fats rather than sugar, margarine, low-fiber diets, vitamin and mineral deficiencies or the proliferation of television sets? Scientists blamed animal fats because these fats tended to increase the serum cholesterol level; however, even those who argue that animal fats are dangerous admit that their effect on serum cholesterol is relatively small.

The third observation, that atherosclerotic plaques contain cholesterol, doesn't really support the lipid hypothesis, either. Studies have shown that most of the cholesterol in arterial plaques doesn't come from the bloodstream but is manufactured from smaller molecules inside the arterial cells. The concept that cholesterol travels from food to the blood and then sticks to the arteries like chewing gum just isn't borne out by our current understanding.

The fourth observation, that feeding cholesterol to animals produces fatty deposits in their arteries, is also incorrect. Cholesterol is an unstable molecule, so much so that mere contact with oxygen in room air causes important changes in its chemical structure. These oxidized cholesterol molecules are extremely toxic; even in minute quantities, they have produced atherosclerosis in animals. Pure cholesterol, on the other hand, didn't produce atherosclerosis, even when fed in large amounts.[6] It's not the cholesterol per se but its toxic by-products that produce atherosclerosis.

This distinction is not just academic. Cholesterol by-products promote plaque buildup not by sticking to the artery wall but by damaging it. Most scientists now agree that injury to the artery is the first and necessary step in the chain of events that lead to hardening of the arteries. Just about any substance that injures blood vessels can promote atherosclerosis. If we are to win the battle against heart disease, we must think in terms of angiotoxins (substances that damage the blood vessels) in general, rather than oxidized cholesterol specifically.

While the lipid hypothesis has been falling out of favor, scientists have been developing a new understanding of how cardiovascular disease occurs. The complex events that lead to a heart attack are now known to be related to more than just atherosclerosis; the behavior of blood platelets and the metabolic efficiency of the heart muscle itself are also important factors. With this new understanding, it has become apparent that vitamin B_6 plays a key role in the prevention and treatment of cardiovascular disease. Not only does this vitamin help prevent atherosclerosis, it also regulates the activity of blood platelets and helps maintain efficient myocardial metabolism.

The Resistance Builder

As I mentioned earlier, damage to blood vessel walls is the first step that leads to atherosclerosis, so one way to prevent hardening of the arteries would be to discover the most important angiotoxins in our diet and our environment and to stay away from them. Another approach would be to strengthen the ability of our blood vessels to resist the damaging effects of these angiotoxins. There is reason to believe that vitamin B_6 might help us accomplish this and so might help prevent atherosclerosis.

Vitamin B_6 is a cofactor for the enzyme called lysyl oxidase.[7] This enzyme keeps blood vessel walls strong by cross-linking amino acids from different protein strands, much as a weaver weaves cloth from individual threads. With insufficient vitamin B_6, lysyl oxidase fails to function properly, and blood vessels become vulnerable to stress and injury.[8]

Atherosclerosis does indeed occur, at least in animals, as a result of B_6 deficiency. James F. Rinehart, M.D., and Louis D. Greenberg, Ph.D., studied the effect on rhesus monkeys of a diet low in B_6. After about five or six months, these animals developed abnormalities in their blood vessels that appeared strikingly similar to human atherosclerosis.[9] This finding was important for two reasons: First, monkeys are close to humans on the evolutionary scale, so the results are more likely to apply to humans than if some other species had been studied. Second, it's unusual for scientists to produce in animals experimental lesions that resemble human atherosclerosis.

The monkey experiment strongly suggests that B_6 deficiency is one of the factors promoting atherosclerosis in humans. Many Americans consume less than the Recommended Dietary Allowance (RDA) for B_6. It's likely that this marginal intake of B_6 over a period of years accelerates the progression of atherosclerosis. Even if we did consume the RDA for B_6 each day, we would have no guarantee that our blood vessels were getting enough of this vitamin. The RDA's were determined by the National Academy of Sciences on the basis of short-term experiments. While 2 milligrams of B_6 a day will prevent acute deficiency, we don't know how much is needed to prevent a disease like atherosclerosis, which takes 30 or more years to develop.

Keeping Platelets in Check

Vitamin B_6 not only maintains the strength of blood vessels, it may also prevent cardiovascular disease by influencing the behavior of blood platelets. There are at least two ways that platelets can affect the heart and blood vessels: First, as they repair damaged blood vessels, platelets release certain chemicals that trigger the formation of plaques. Second, platelets appear to promote blood vessel spasms. One of the chemicals that platelets release when they aggregate is called thromboxane. This chemical can indirectly cause blood vessels to contract, reducing blood flow and causing angina or infarction. This sequence of events can be prevented by substances that inhibit platelets from aggregating. Studies have shown that when pyridoxal phosphate (the biologically active form of B_6) is added to a test tube, it inhibits the tendency of platelets to clump together. When human volunteers ingested 100 milligrams of pyridoxine, their platelet function was blocked for up to 52 hours.[10] By inhibiting platelets, vitamin B_6 might therefore prevent both atherosclerosis and blood vessel spasm.

On June 13, 1981, an editorial appeared in the prestigious British journal *Lancet*, titled "Is Vitamin B_6 an Antithrombotic Agent?"[11] This editorial reviewed a number of studies demonstrating that B_6 inhibits blood from clotting not only by interfering with platelet function but also by blocking the clotting activity of thrombin (another molecule involved in blood clotting). The authors of this review suggested that "moderate doses of vitamin B$_6$ (say, 40 milligrams a day) may suffice to alter the natural history" of cardiovascular disease. Biochemists from the University of Toronto have echoed this opinion, pointing out that the effect of B$_6$ on thrombin may turn out to be more important than its effects on platelets.[12]

We will see throughout this book that vitamin B$_6$ and magnesium work together in a number of different biochemical systems. Many B$_6$-dependent enzymes also require magnesium for normal activity, and without adequate vitamin B$_6$, magnesium has difficulty traveling from the blood or fluid surrounding cells into the cells themselves. Like B$_6$, magnesium prevents platelet aggregation. Magnesium also prevents coronary artery spasms and can normalize certain dangerous cardiac rhythm disturbances. In addition, magnesium injections have produced dramatic relief in patients with angina pectoris (chest pain associated with heart disease) after all other treatments had failed and the patients had lost all hope of recovery. In two other studies done in the 1950's, magnesium injections reduced the death rate in cardiac patients by more than 90 percent![5] Because vitamin B$_6$ and magnesium work so well together, they should be an effective team in the battle against heart disease.

A Healthy Heart Muscle

Scientists have only recently begun to recognize how large a role myocardial metabolism plays in cardiovascular health. A heart that is an efficient biochemical machine can get by with less oxygen than a poorly functioning heart. Nutrients needed for energy production, such as vitamin B$_6$ and magnesium, would therefore increase the heart's resistance to atherosclerosis. In one study, rats fed a diet low in B$_6$ developed abnormally large hearts (often an indication that the heart is not functioning properly).[13] In another experiment with rats, vitamin B$_6$ deficiency resulted in the kind of abnormal changes in the electrocardiogram that indicate heart disease.[14]

Studies in Humans

It's time that we begin intensive research *with human beings* to determine the best ways to use vitamin B$_6$ to prevent and treat cardiovascular disease. As with many other promising nutritional remedies, B_6 has largely been ignored by traditional doctors. Instead, they prefer to use potentially toxic drugs to inhibit platelet aggregation and prevent vasospasm. Only John M. Ellis, M.D., a pioneer in vitamin B_6 therapy, has used this vitamin extensively in heart patients and reported his findings.[15] Dr. Ellis routinely gave an intramuscular injection of 100 milligrams of B_6 to patients who were being hospitalized for suspected myocardial infarction. He found that electrocardiograms of those who received the vitamin showed less deviation (possibly indicative of less heart damage) than patients who had not been given the injection. Dr. Ellis also noted that the edema (swelling) associated with heart disease could be partly relieved by vitamin B_6.

Because he was a family doctor trying to give his patients the best possible treatment, Dr. Ellis was not in a position to do a controlled study. Skeptics might therefore wish to reserve judgment on vitamin B_6 therapy until it has been studied more fully. Unfortunately, the demands imposed by the scientific method have placed nutrition-oriented physicians and their patients in something of a Catch-22. We are told that vitamin B_6 therapy (and other nutritional treatments) should be considered experimental until we can come up with placebo-controlled, double-blind studies. The problem is that these expensive and rigorous studies can't possibly be performed by the typical practitioner in the community. Only doctors at large research centers can obtain the funds and the technical support required to prove that something works. Sadly, these doctors are often the same ones that criticize nutrition data as being "soft" and have no interest in pursuing potentially important discoveries made by outsiders.

The results Dr. Ellis obtained are sufficiently encouraging to demand urgent follow-up by research centers, however. The profoundly important work on magnesium that lies buried in medical journals published three decades ago also needs to be revived.

It's time for our scientists to compare the effects of B_6 and magnesium with those of the currently used platelet-inhibiting drugs (aspirin, dipyridamole, sulphinpyrazone, etc.). B_6 may yet turn out to be more effective than any of the antiplatelet drugs yet tested, since it is one of the few compounds that inhibits blood coagulation in two separate ways. It is also time that the calcium channel blockers (nifedipine, verapamil, and others) currently used to prevent vasospasm, be compared with the combined effects of magnesium and vitamin B_6. I wouldn't be surprised to find that these nutrients, properly administered, work better and cause fewer side effects than the drugs.

What You Can Do Now

Until the necessary research is done, any decisions you make concerning nutritional therapy must be based on limited information. This isn't to say that you should delay every decision you make about diet and supplements until all the research is in. From what we already know, it's possible to devise a sensible nutritional approach to heart disease that is unlikely to cause harm and might provide considerable benefit.

Prudence dictates that you minimize your intake of refined sugar, hydrogenated oil and overheated vegetable oil. Numerous studies that are beyond the scope of this book suggest that these foods promote cardiovascular disease. Animal fats should also be used in moderation, and special care should be taken to avoid oxidized cholesterol. For example, a scrambled egg might be considerably more hazardous than one boiled in its shell. Processed food and salt should also be used prudently.

Nutritional supplements, particularly magnesium and vitamin B_6, may ultimately be proved to reduce the incidence of cardiovascular disease. Even though the final word is not yet in, it would not be unreasonable for you, with your doctor's approval, to supplement your diet with these nutrients.

Preliminary studies also suggest a role for vitamins C and E, niacin, pantothenate, calcium, zinc, copper, chromium, selenium (in limited amounts) and silicon in the prevention and treatment of heart disease. If we would combine what we are learning about nutrition with an extensive effort to rid our environment of angiotoxic substances, we might soon find ourselves nearing the answer to the riddle of heart disease.

Chapter

Cancer 8

Cancer is a leading cause of death in the United States, second only to heart disease. The incidence of this dreaded illness has increased steadily during the twentieth century. If present trends continue, about one out of every four Americans will eventually develop some type of malignancy.

The mere mention of the word *cancer* almost always triggers an emotional reaction. The thought of foreign cells growing uncontrollably inside one's body, the anticipation of wasting away while suffering severe pain, and the sense of hopelessness that comes with the diagnosis makes cancer the most dreaded of all diseases. Fewer than 15 percent of those with cancer of the esophagus, stomach, pancreas or lung will be alive five years after their disease is diagnosed. The survival rate for other types of cancer, though somewhat better, is also unacceptably low.

Many cancer victims live out the last years of their lives in despair and agony. In addition to the toll taken by the disease itself, cancer victims must also face the demoralizing and uncomfortable side effects of modern treatment. In an attempt to control their pain, cancer patients often become dependent on narcotics, which dull the senses and can produce unrelenting constipation. Chemotherapy often causes nausea, vomiting and hair loss, and may suppress the immune system so that even the simplest infection can land the cancer victim in the hospital. Radiation therapy often produces some of these side effects, too, and surgical removal of a tumor can disfigure the patient or weaken the immune system.

Some people feel that the ordeals of these treatments hardly seem worth their benefits, since statistics show that many cancer patients do not survive much longer now than they did 25 years ago. Although results with some of the less common types of cancer—childhood leukemia, Hodgkin's disease and testicular tumors—are encouraging, the figures for the more common cancers—breast, colon, lung, pancreas, bladder, prostate, rectum and cervix—remain grim.[1] Many authorities now believe that the war against cancer will not be won by developing more powerful chemotherapy and radiation or more-radical surgical procedures. Rather, the key to cancer control will be found in (1) identifying and avoiding cancer-causing agents, and (2) bolstering the body's natural ability to fight cancer at an early stage of the disease.

Bolstering Immunity

Because of its ability to stimulate the immune system, vitamin B_6 may be one important link in the chain of cancer prevention and treatment. It's now well accepted that the body's immune system plays a major role in defending against malignant cells. Composed of an intricate network of white blood cells and specialized tissues in the spleen, lymph nodes, thymus, liver and elsewhere, the immune system hunts down and destroys foreign cells. Scientists now agree that normal cells have a continuous tendency to become transformed into malignant cells, but as long as the "immune surveillance" mechanism is operating, these newly formed malignant cells will be detected and destroyed before they've had a chance to multiply. If the immune system becomes impaired, some of these transformed cells will multiply and eventually invade the rest of the body.

Vitamin B_6 helps promote a healthy immune system in a number of ways.[2,3] Animal experiments have shown that white blood cells need B_6 to manufacture antibodies. In addition, the thymus gland, an important component of the immune system, can't function properly without adequate B_6. This vitamin is also necessary for the white blood cells known as lymphocytes to perform their usual "search-and-destroy" missions.

Bladder Cancer Studies

Vitamin B_6 may be especially important in people suffering from bladder cancer, because it appears to control the metabolism of tryptophan, an amino acid. With enough B_6, the body can convert tryptophan into relatively harmless or even beneficial compounds, such as niacin. But if B_6 is lacking, the body may convert tryptophan into various carcinogens, such as 3-hydroxy-L-kynurenine (3-OH-K), 3-hydroxyanthranilic acid (3-OH-AA) and xanthurenic acid (XA)—all of which are believed to cause bladder cancer.

A study conducted by scientists at the University of Wisconsin suggests that susceptibility to bladder cancer depends in part on how a person's body metabolizes tryptophan.[4] The scientists implanted small pellets containing 3-OH-K, 3-OH-AA and XA into the bladders of mice, and each of these pellets produced bladder cancer. Next, the scientists studied tryptophan metabolism in 38 people with bladder cancer.[5] Eighteen of the 38 excreted large amounts of the compounds that had caused bladder cancer in mice, and everyone in the group had a recurrence of bladder cancer within five years. The remaining 20 had normal tryptophan metabolism; of this group, only 12 had a recurrence within five years. On the basis of this evidence, it's logical to assume that since B_6 is capable of shifting tryptophan metabolism away from the cancer-causing compounds, supplements of the vitamin might help prevent bladder cancer in some cases.

Clinical Evidence

Theories based solely on biochemical observations don't always apply in real life. Although the connection between B_6 and bladder cancer is still unproven, it has been carefully tested in a controlled clinical trial, with promising results.[6]

David Byar, M.D., and Clyde Blackard, M.D., have reported a study by the Veterans Administration Cooperative Urological Research Group, in which they recruited 121 patients with bladder cancer from a dozen Veterans Administration hospitals around the United States. Each patient was given one of three treatments: (1) pyridoxine (B_6), 25 milligrams a day; (2) thiotepa, a drug frequently used to treat bladder cancer; or (3) a placebo. The study was designed to last two years;

however, for various reasons, some patients dropped out before this time. By the end of the study, bladder tumors had recurred in 47 percent of those treated with B_6. This recurrence rate was the same as that among the patients given the standard treatment (thiotepa). The patients treated with the placebo fared somewhat worse: More than 60 percent developed a new tumor during the study. The difference between vitamin B_6 and the placebo wasn't statistically significant; in other words, the results in the B_6 group could have been due to chance. (Of course, so could the results in the drug group.)

Despite the lack of firm proof, this study suggested that some patients had indeed benefited from vitamin B_6 treatment. Drs. Byar and Blackard considered the possibility that B_6's elimination of cancer-causing molecules from the urine might have a delayed effect. To check this possibility, they divided their patients into two groups: (1) those who had a recurrence of cancer or who dropped out of the study during the first ten months, and (2) those who remained free of cancer during these ten months. When the second group alone was considered, vitamin B_6 treatment was found to be significantly better than placebo therapy. In other words, vitamin B_6 therapy reduced the subsequent recurrence rate.[6]

For rather complicated reasons, some statisticians would argue that Drs. Byar and Blackard should not have divided their patients into subgroups once the study had already been completed. This means that we cannot consider the benefits of B_6 in bladder cancer to be scientifically proved. The work of these researchers is quite promising, however, and should be followed up. Further research could determine which people are most likely to benefit from B_6 therapy. Not all victims of this disease have abnormal tryptophan metabolism.[7] Would only those who excrete the "wrong" tryptophan by-products benefit? Would higher doses of B_6 work better than the 25 milligrams a day studied by Drs. Byar and Blackard? Because vitamin B_6 is so safe and inexpensive compared to the drugs used to treat cancer, answers to these questions are urgently needed.

Until all the answers are in, it seems reasonable to recommend that all people suffering from bladder cancer take at least 25 milligrams of B_6 a day. This dose is quite safe, and it may turn out to be helpful. Doctors should measure tryptophan metabolites in all patients who have bladder cancer. Without such studies, there is no way to determine how much B_6 is needed to keep the cancer-causing tryptophan metabolites out of the urine. It's likely that the optimal dose of B_6 varies from person to person. Perhaps some people with bladder cancer have a hereditary abnormality of tryptophan metabolism, requiring larger-than-normal amounts of B_6.

Further Evidence

Whether or not vitamin B_6 supplements prevent bladder cancer from developing in the first place is not known. From what we do know about tryptophan, vitamin B_6 and bladder cancer, it wouldn't be surprising to discover that this vitamin has a preventive effect. Several additional pieces of circumstantial evidence support this view. First, there is an increased risk of bladder cancer in people who have been treated for tuberculosis with the drug isoniazid (INH).[8] This drug is a B_6 antimetabolite. Some people who take INH even develop neuritis because of severe B_6 deficiency. In studies where animals were given INH, their urinary excretion of xanthurenic acid increased.[9] As you may recall, xanthurenic acid is an abnormal by-product of tryptophan metabolism that is produced when vitamin B_6 is lacking. Furthermore, xanthurenic acid causes bladder cancer in animals. The fact that INH causes B_6 deficiency and may also promote bladder tumors supports the concept that B_6 helps prevent such tumors.

Another important bit of circumstantial evidence is that smokers have a relatively high risk of developing bladder cancer.[8] As I mentioned in chapter 1, tobacco smoke contains traces of hydrazine and maleic hydrazide, both of which may be vitamin B_6 antimetabolites. These chemicals and a host of other hydrazines and hydrazides cause cancer in animals.[10] Most of these compounds are also known or suspected vitamin B_6 antagonists. Do hydrazines and hydrazides promote cancer by interfering with the function of B_6? Would vitamin B_6 supplements prevent the tendency of these toxins to cause cancer?

We might also ask whether other cancer-causing substances produce their damage by interfering with B_6 metabolism. Some edible mushrooms contain hydrazine compounds, which are both cancer-causing agents and suspected vitamin B_6 antagonists.[10] Animal studies have shown that heat can turn some of the chemicals in vegetable oils into powerful carcinogens.[11] Heated vegetable oils also contain by-products that increase the need for vitamin B_6. If eating heated vegetable oil does increase our risk of cancer, can we reduce this risk by taking more vitamin B_6?

As you can see, much remains to be learned about vitamin B_6 and its relationship to cancer. What dose of this vitamin is most likely to be beneficial? Can we minimize the dangers of our carcinogenic environment by taking more B_6? Is there a way to identify people who are especially sensitive to B_6 antimetabolites? Would they need larger amounts of B_6 to help fight cancer? The list of questions is seemingly endless.

We will ultimately conquer cancer not by developing more-powerful toxic drugs, but by devising more-effective ways to stimulate the body's own defenses. The use of certain vitamins and minerals to prevent and treat cancer is beginning to look quite promising. There is growing awareness that selenium, vitamins A, C and E, beta carotene and other nutrients can be used safely and effectively in the battle against cancer.

It's imperative that these preliminary findings be followed up and expanded upon. It is time for a new orientation in cancer research. We can no longer afford to waste research money and valuable time pursuing toxic treatments that have produced few worthwhile results. Unfortunately, certain special interests would be threatened by a well-funded, intense study of nutrition and cancer. If we could somehow cut through these conflicts of interest and direct research funding where it belongs, then the cure of this dread disease might perhaps be just around the corner.

Chapter
Diabetes 9

Diabetes, a disorder in which the body has difficulty metabolizing carbohydrates, has become increasingly prevalent in the United States over the past several decades. As many as 10 million Americans now suffer from diabetes, and this number will probably continue to rise. Diabetes and its complications are currently the fifth leading cause of death in the United States.

The term *diabetes* is actually short for diabetes mellitus, which is derived from Greek. *Diabetes* means "to run through," referring to the profuse urination that is a hallmark of the disease. *Mellitus* means "sweet." The full name describes the large volume of sweet urine that results when glucose spills from the blood into the urine. The abbreviated name diabetes is not strictly correct, because the word can also refer to diabetes insipidus, another disorder, in which an abnormal pituitary gland causes voluminous urination. Since diabetes insipidus is extremely rare and diabetes mellitus is common, we generally use the term *diabetes* to indicate the latter.

The basic abnormality in diabetes is the way the body handles glucose. In normal people, starches and sugars in the diet are converted to the simple sugar glucose, which is then transported across the intestinal wall and into the bloodstream. Under the direction of the pancreatic hormone insulin, glucose travels from the blood into the cells of the body, where it's used to produce energy. Diabetics have difficulty transporting glucose into their cells. As a result, their blood sugar level remains elevated, but their cells are starved for fuel.

Diabetes can be caused by either insulin deficiency or insulin resistance. Normally, insulin manufactured in the pancreas is secreted into the blood after a meal. This hormone somehow stimulates the cells to take up glucose. In diabetics, however, this insulin mechanism fails. In some cases, the pancreas produces too little insulin or none at all. More commonly, a normal or increased amount of insulin is present, but the cells are unable to process the message transmitted by this hormone. This breakdown in communication is called "insulin resistance."

Because diabetics have difficulty handling glucose, one of the most fundamental molecules in the body, all sorts of things tend to go wrong with their metabolism. As their blood glucose level rises, some of this sugar spills into the urine, drawing additional water along with it by osmosis. With large glucose spills, the water loss can lead to dehydration.

A far more serious complication of diabetes is ketoacidosis, a dangerous shift in the body's acid/base balance that takes place when the cells can't get enough glucose and have to resort to burning fat for energy. When fat breaks down, it yields several highly acidic compounds called ketones. The more ketones produced, the more acidic the body becomes. The combination of ketoacidosis and dehydration is a life-threatening medical emergency.

Fortunately, with diet modification, nutritional supplements and therapy with insulin or other medications, most diabetics are able to avoid slipping into ketoacidosis or becoming severely dehydrated. Even with usual therapy, however, many diabetics eventually develop other complications. Over the years the continued biochemical stress created by impaired glucose metabolism can take its toll in a number of different ways. Damage to the retina of the eye (retinopathy) is one common complication that can lead to blindness. Impaired nervous system function (neuropathy) is another complication. Its symptoms include numbness, tingling, pain or loss of sensation in the extremities, weakness, paralysis, sexual impotence, urinary difficulties, low blood pressure and digestive disturbances. The kidneys may also succumb to diabetes, necessitating dialysis in some cases. The risk of cardiovascular disease is also about twice as high in diabetics as in the general population. In addition, diabetics are prone to infections of all types, including urinary tract infections and difficult-to-treat yeast infections.

A special problem that diabetics must contend with is ulceration of the skin on the toes, feet or legs. These ulcers tend to become easily infected and, if not carefully treated, may lead to gangrene. Ulcers cause problems in diabetics because they tend to have poor circulation due to atherosclerosis (hardening of the arteries). This means that not enough blood reaches the legs and feet to promote healing or fight infections. Many diabetics can't care for their ulcers properly because retinopathy may have impaired their vision and neuropathy may have decreased their sensitivity to pain. A simple cut or scrape between the toes or on the foot may simply go unnoticed until it has become so infected that an arterial bypass operation is needed to halt the progression of gangrene. When bypass surgery is too risky or unsuccessful, amputation may be necessary. Forty percent of amputations are performed on diabetics with life-threatening gangrene. Unfortunately, after amputation of a leg, as many as one-third of diabetics have to have the other leg removed within three years.

Studies have shown that controlling glucose levels by strict diets and closely monitored insulin injections can slow down nerve damage and improve kidney and retinal damage.[1,2] That's why it's so important for diabetics to try to keep their blood sugar as close to normal as possible at all times.

One of the best ways for the diabetic to control blood sugar is through careful diet. More than half a dozen studies over the past several years have shown that a diet low in refined sugar, containing large amounts of whole grains, dried beans, fresh vegetables and other high-fiber foods will lower the blood sugar in many cases.[3,4] Apparently, high-fiber foods prevent large rises in blood sugar because these foods are absorbed more slowly and more evenly than other foods. Several studies have documented the ability of brewer's yeast to lower blood sugar in diabetics.[5,6] This widely used nutritional supplement is a rich source of a chromium-containing molecule called glucose tolerance factor, which helps keep the blood sugar down by allowing the body's insulin to perform more efficiently. Medical nutritionists frequently recommend other supplements for diabetics, including B-complex vitamins, vitamins C and E, magnesium, zinc, copper, chromium, manganese, thyroid hormone and garlic.

Carbohydrate metabolism is extremely complex; a host of different vitamins, minerals and hormones are involved in the regulation of blood sugar. No single nutritional supplement should be expected to solve the problem of diabetes. Still, a well-formulated program of diet and nutritional supplements will often lower blood sugar and reduce the need for insulin injections. Lowering the insulin requirement is a worthwhile goal in its own right, in view of evidence that insulin itself may accelerate atherosclerosis.[7]

Vitamin B_6 supplements may be helpful for diabetics for several reasons. Although this vitamin alone will obviously not cure diabetes, it may play a role in keeping the blood sugar level down. More important, B_6 may be able to prevent or reverse some of the complications of diabetes.

Richard E. Davis, M.D., and colleagues at the University of Western Australia have found that some diabetics tend to be low in vitamin B_6. Dr. Davis measured the level of pyridoxal (one of the forms of vitamin B_6) in the serum of 518 diabetics and found that 25 percent were B_6 deficient.[8] This deficiency was unrelated to what the diabetics were eating, or to whether they were taking insulin or other antidiabetic medications. Dr. Davis concluded that diabetics may have a higher-than-average need for vitamin B_6.

Improving Glucose Tolerance

There is some evidence that vitamin B_6 deficiency leads to impaired glucose tolerance or worsening of diabetes. In two studies, vitamin B_6 supplements were found to improve glucose tolerance.[9,10] As I mentioned in chapter 3, B_6 has also been used with some success in treating gestational diabetes (the diabetes that sometimes accompanies pregnancy). In addition, B_6 can improve the abnormal glucose tolerance that develops in some women who take birth control pills.[11,12] In another study, however, vitamin B_6 supplements had no effect on the glucose metabolism of 13 diabetics.[13]

The question of whether B_6 improves glucose metabolism should be studied further, but the research done so far suggests that B_6 supplements will help improve glucose tolerance in some cases of diabetes. Since diabetics as a group tend to be low in this vitamin, and since B_6 therapy is safe and inexpensive, it is not unreasonable to suggest that all diabetics (with their doctor's approval) take additional B_6.

If vitamin B_6 does improve glucose tolerance, how does it work? There is some evidence that the effect of B_6 is related to xanthurenic acid (XA), a by-product of tryptophan metabolism. As I mentioned in chapter 1, B_6-deficient people have certain abnormalities in their tryptophan metabolism that lead to the production of excess XA. This tryptophan by-product possesses the interesting (though possibly dangerous) property of being able to bind onto insulin and inactivate it.[14] Theoretically, B_6 supplements should improve glucose tolerance by reducing XA production. Some scientists have questioned this explanation of how B_6 improves glucose tolerance. At this point, all we know is that B_6 appears to aid some diabetics, but we're not sure why.

Because B_6 appears to improve glucose tolerance in at least some cases, this vitamin may help prevent the long-term complications of diabetes. As I mentioned, controlling blood sugar is a good way to reduce the chance of typical kidney, nerve, eye or blood vessel complications. However, even if B_6 had nothing to do with glucose metabolism, there would still be several good reasons that diabetics should take additional quantities of this vitamin. Specifically, vitamin B_6 may, in ways that are unrelated to glucose metabolism, prevent the diabetic from developing neuropathy, infections and hardening of the arteries.

Curing Neuropathy

Some tuberculosis patients whose isoniazid therapy caused their B_6 levels to fall have developed symptoms that resemble diabetic neuropathy. Because diabetics are often low in B_6, it's possible that diabetic neuropathy is partly due to B_6 deficiency. Dr. Davis measured vitamin B_6 in the serum of a group of diabetics. He found that B_6 levels were significantly lower in people who suffered from neuropathy than in those who didn't.[15] Perhaps B_6 supplements could prevent or relieve diabetic neuropathy.

Charles L. Jones, D.P.M., a podiatrist, and Virgilio Gonzalez, M.D.,[16] studied ten insulin-dependent diabetics who had symptoms of peripheral neuropathy (neuropathy outside the central nervous system). These patients excreted more xanthurenic acid than did other diabetics without neuropathy, suggesting that B_6 deficiency was more pronounced in the patients suffering from neuropathy. When Drs. Jones and Gonzalez gave each patient 50 milligrams of pyridoxine three times a day for six weeks, xanthurenic acid excretion became normal, indicating that B_6 deficiency had been corrected. And, even more important, symptoms of neuropathy disappeared in all ten patients. Most of them noticed some relief of pain and paresthesia (abnormal sensation) in about ten days. This improvement continued and became even more pronounced as the study progressed. Every one of the patients also remarked that their eyes "felt better," a benefit that had not been anticipated by the researchers.

Seven of the patients continued on B_6 supplements and did well. The other three stopped taking the vitamin and noticed a recurrence of their symptoms about three weeks later. When they resumed taking B_6, their symptoms again disappeared. Two patients in the study also had a marked improvement in their blood sugar measurements, which had been chronically elevated (275 and 315 milligrams per hundred milliliters, respectively) and difficult to control. After B_6 therapy, their glucose levels fell to 195 and 200, respectively, and remained there as long as they continued taking B_6.

The work of Drs. Jones and Gonzalez is an important advance in the treatment of diabetes. Neuropathy is an annoying and painful complication of diabetes, which can increase the risk of infection, ulceration, injury or gangrene. Standard drug treatment for neuropathy is potentially dangerous and often ineffective.

Another group of investigators, stimulated by the work of Drs. Jones and Gonzalez, also tried vitamin B_6 in 18 diabetic patients with peripheral neuropathy. In this study, half the patients were treated with a placebo to eliminate the possibility that improvements were due to psychological factors. After four months, 6 of the 9 patients taking pyridoxine (50 milligrams three times a day) noted significant relief of their symptoms. Four of the 9 placebo-treated patients experienced similar benefits. The difference between vitamin B_6 and the placebo was not statistically significant. In other words, the better results with B_6 could have occurred by chance. The scientists, headed by Ellis R. Levin, M.D., concluded that vitamin B_6 deficiency is probably not a factor in diabetic peripheral neuropathy, since a "similar" percentage of individuals improved in each group.[17]

The conclusions of Dr. Levin's group are unwarranted. Sixty-seven percent and 44 percent can hardly be considered "similar." The fact that some people improved while taking a placebo does not change the fact that more patients improved with B_6 therapy. If this group had found similar results with two groups of 900, rather than two groups of 9 patients, then the results would have been much more impressive (and statistically significant). Six hundred sixty-seven diabetics would have improved from B_6 compared with only 444 from placebo. These scientists made a common error because they did not understand the meaning of their statistics. (See chapter 5 for further discussion of this point.) The correct interpretation of their study is as follows: "Vitamin B_6 was more effective than the placebo in relieving diabetic neuropathy; however, there is at least a 5 percent probability that these results are due to chance."

It's wrong to conclude that B_6 is ineffective merely because there is some chance it is ineffective. Until a larger study is done, all that can be said is that B_6 looks promising. I have had a number of diabetic patients whose numbness and pain in their extremities improved while they were taking B_6. Others did not seem to benefit, but did improve after a course of vitamin B_{12} injections. Still others found no relief from any treatment. As with other common disorders, diabetic neuropathy probably has several different causes, of which abnormal vitamin B_6 and vitamin B_{12} metabolism[18,19] appear to be two.

No single treatment will be effective for everyone; however, if a remedy is safe and inexpensive, and if it holds some possibility of success, it shouldn't be rejected merely because final proof is not yet in. As our knowledge continues to advance, we will become more adept at predicting who is most likely to improve from which treatments. In the meantime, nutrition-oriented physicians continue to make educated guesses, often with gratifying results.

Increased resistance against infections is another B_6 bonus for diabetics. Vitamin B_6 deficiency might be one reason that diabetics are so infection-prone, since adequate amounts of this vitamin are needed for the immune system to function properly. Dr. Davis has reported that diabetics with urinary tract infections had less B_6 in their blood than did other diabetics.[20] This reduction in B_6 levels was not due to the infection itself, because the deficiency persisted for at least six months after treatment cleared up the infection. Again, B_6 supplements may not solve the problem completely, but any safe treatment that might help prevent infections in diabetics is welcomed.

Diabetics are about twice as likely as others to be affected by hardening of the arteries and heart attacks. As we've seen in chapter 7, vitamin B_6 supplements seem to play an important role in preventing these common and serious illnesses.

As always, you should consult your doctor before taking nutritional supplements. With diabetes in particular, unsupervised use of vitamins and minerals can be risky. Some nutrients, including vitamin B_6, will lower the blood sugar in certain people. While this change is beneficial in the long run, it may cause dangerous low blood sugar reactions in people taking insulin or other medication for diabetes. On the other hand, if your blood sugar is monitored appropriately, there should be little danger in trying vitamin B_6. In fact it might turn out to be quite helpful.

Chapter

Systemic 10
Lupus
Erythematosus

Systemic lupus erythematosus (SLE) is a serious and often fatal autoimmune disease in which the body's immune system attacks it own tissues. This disease affects an estimated 60,000 to 740,000 Americans.[1] The word *lupus* is derived from Latin and means "wolf." *Erythematosus* denotes redness. Together the terms describe this disease, in which reddened lesions resembling a wolf bite appear on the face. Two different syndromes are called lupus erythematosus, or LE: discoid LE affects only the skin and is not life-threatening or serious. The subject of this chapter is the systemic form of this disorder, known as SLE.

No one knows what causes SLE. It affects many different organs and tissues and tends to come and go unpredictably. There is no single textbook description of SLE, but the syndrome does have certain common characteristics. Many patients experience fever, weight loss and arthritic symptoms resembling rheumatoid arthritis. These may be accompanied by cardiac problems, including cardiomegaly (enlarged heart), myocarditis or pericarditis (inflammation of the heart muscle or the sac surrounding the heart, respectively), heart failure, electrocardiographic changes, heart murmurs or high blood pressure. The lungs may also be affected, resulting in pleurisy or pleural effusion (inflammation of, or fluid buildup in, the sac surrounding the lungs, respectively) or pneumonia, which can be fatal. The disease may also cause hives, hair loss and purpura (purple spots that resemble bruises). Many patients with SLE become photosensitive (i.e., their skin problems may worsen after sun exposure). When the central nervous system is afflicted, partial paralysis, convulsions, neuritis or severe psychiatric illness may result. Sometimes the nervous system damage is fatal. If SLE hits the gastrointestinal tract, it may cause nausea, vomiting, diarrhea, ulcerative colitis or jaundice. Abnormalities of the blood, such as anemia or low platelet counts, are not uncommon. Low white blood cell counts might predispose the patient to serious infections. SLE tends to attack the kidneys as well, sometimes causing death from kidney failure.

Normally, our immune system protects us against bacteria, viruses, foreign chemicals and other unwanted invaders. A complicated and powerful network of white blood cells works in concert with the liver, spleen and lungs to engulf and destroy these invaders. The immune system defends us against a hostile environment; when our immune systems fail, we can die from even the most innocent infections.

For reasons still unknown to science, the immune system is not always able to distinguish the body's own tissues from those of foreign invaders. When this happens, the same mechanisms that protect us from our environment can damage our own organs and tissues. This is what happens in SLE.

The Symptom Masquerade

Before the discovery of cortisonelike drugs, victims of SLE usually died within several years of diagnosis. These drugs and new treatment approaches have improved the outlook. Still, only about 50 or 60 percent of SLE sufferers will be alive ten years after being diagnosed,[2] and SLE seems to be on the rise. In 1928 not a single patient was admitted to the Los Angeles County General Hospital with a diagnosis of SLE, but by 1948 the hospital was admitting 9 cases a year, and by 1962, it was admitting an average of 66 patients with this disorder each year. Some scientists have argued that SLE is not really more common but that doctors are simply diagnosing it more. Since SLE's symptoms can masquerade as some other disease, many cases of SLE have been improperly classified. Before the antibiotic era, some patients may have died of an infection before their other symptoms became severe enough to suggest an SLE diagnosis. Before 1948, no specific test for SLE had been developed, and many cases of SLE were classified as atypical rheumatoid arthritis, for example. Despite the difficulties of comparing today's statistics with those of past years, some investigators believe the disease is truly becoming more prevalent.[1]

Perhaps the rising incidence of B_6 deficiency is partly to blame for the increase in SLE. Several bits of circumstantial evidence suggest that B_6 deficiency may play a role in this disease. Although the proposed relationship between vitamin B_6 and SLE is purely hypothetical, circumstantial evidence often provides the foundation for definitive research.

A Drug-Induced Version

For many years we have known that certain drugs can produce side effects that closely resemble SLE. This syndrome is termed drug-induced lupus.[3] The main differences between SLE and its drug-induced counterpart are that kidney disease is rare in drug-induced lupus and some diagnostic tests give different results than in SLE. Also, drug-induced lupus usually disappears once the offending drug is discontinued.

At least 20 medications have been reported to cause drug-induced lupus. Most of these drugs differ in chemical structure and clinical use, but a good percentage contain either hydrazine or hydrazide molecules, inhibit vitamin B_6, or both. One such drug is hydralazine, commonly used to treat high blood pressure and congestive heart failure. This drug is a hydrazine compound, and it produces B_6 deficiency[4] as well as causing drug-induced lupus. Phenelzine is another hydrazine compound that has been reported to produce a lupuslike reaction in at least one patient.[5] Used to treat depression, phenelzine is also known to inhibit vitamin B_6.[4] Drug-induced lupus has also been attributed to birth control pills. Although the Pill does not have a hydrazine structure, it is a well-documented cause of vitamin B_6 deficiency.[6] Isoniazid (INH) is a hydrazide compound prescribed for the prevention and treatment of tuberculosis. It, too, is a well-known cause of B_6 deficiency[7] and has been reported to trigger a lupuslike syndrome. Penicillamine, used to treat rheumatoid arthritis and a disorder of copper metabolism known as Wilson's disease, has also caused drug-induced lupus and has been shown to produce vitamin B_6 deficiency.[4] In fact, nearly all drugs that antagonize vitamin B_6 have been shown to cause lupus.

Do B₆ Antagonists Play a Role?

If medications that interfere with B_6 can induce lupus, perhaps some of the B_6 antagonists present in our environment can do the same (see chapter 1). Do the maleic hydrazide and the succinic acid 2,2-dimethylhydrazide that we spray on our crops contribute to the development of SLE? Is the hydrazine used in rocket fuel and present in tobacco smoke a factor? What about the PCB's used by industry? Do vegetable oils oxidized at high temperatures increase the risk of lupus? Is the annual addition of one million pounds of tartrazine to our food supply important?

These questions cannot be answered without additional research. We must consider the possibility, however, that B_6 antagonists promote SLE. During the past three decades, our exposure to vitamin B_6 antimetabolites has increased profoundly. During this same time, according to some scientists, there has been an increase in the incidence of SLE. There is clearly some relationship among vitamin B_6, hydrazines and lupus, but no one knows exactly what it is. I am not suggesting that hydrazines and/or B_6 deficiency are the *sole* causes of SLE—there are probably many other environmental and hereditary factors as well. I am suggesting, however, that hydrazines and B_6 deficiency may increase an individual's risk of developing lupus.

Prostaglandin Protection

How might vitamin B_6 deficiency promote the development of SLE? The answer to this question must be speculative, because the cause of lupus is still not understood. It's possible, however, that B_6 antagonists interfere with the metabolism of prostaglandins.

Prostaglandins are hormonelike compounds manufactured by the body from essential fatty acids such as linoleic and linolenic acids. There are many different prostaglandins, and they perform many different biochemical functions. The results of animal studies suggest that one of these compounds, prostaglandin E1 (PGE1), may play a role in preventing lupus.

Scientists have studied animals to learn more about what happens in human SLE. When New Zealand black (NZB) mice are bred with New Zealand white (NZW) mice, their offspring are known as NZB/NZW mice. These offspring spontaneously develop a disease that is remarkably similar to SLE in humans. As NZB/NZW mice mature, they develop various signs and symptoms, including autoimmune kidney disease and abnormal blood tests similar to those in human SLE. The mice usually die prematurely from kidney failure.

When a group of NZB/NZW mice were injected with PGE1 once or twice daily between 6 and 52 weeks of age, PGE1 protected them against anemia, kidney disease and premature death. At one year of age, 18 of 19 treated mice were alive, while only 2 of 19 untreated control mice had survived.[8]

David F. Horrobin, M.D., Ph.D., a Canadian researcher, has pointed out that the body may need vitamin B_6 to convert linoleic acid into PGE1.[9] If there is a B_6 deficiency, or if B_6 antagonists are present, the body might not be able to manufacture adequate amounts of PGE1. If this prostaglandin is as important in human lupus as it is in mice, then a B_6 deficiency would increase the risk of developing SLE. Similarly, B_6 antimetabolites might promote lupus by inhibiting the enzyme that produces PGE1.

It's not yet clear how PGE1 might protect against lupus. Dr. Horrobin believes, however, that it acts by stimulating so-called suppressor T-cells. Normally the immune system is endowed with certain "checks and balances" that allow it to destroy foreign invaders without attacking the body's own cells. The prime movers in this system of checks and balances are a group of white blood cells known as suppressor T-cells, so called because they are derived from the thymus gland and they suppress the immune system's tendency to damage friendly tissues.

If the suppressor T-cells are functioning normally, the chance of autoimmune disease is reduced. There is evidence that the suppressor T-cells of most people suffering from SLE don't function normally.[10] As I said, Dr. Horrobin has pointed out that PGE1 is necessary for normal suppressor T-cell function.[9] Perhaps the beneficial effects of PGE1 on NZB/NZW mice are due to stimulation of suppressor T-cells. Whatever the reason, it's clear that PGE1 improves spontaneous lupus in animals. Whether it will also help human lupus sufferers has not yet been determined, but it's certainly an exciting possibility. Because B_6 is apparently necessary for the body to synthesize PGE1, it's possible that B_6 antagonists are a cause of SLE in humans.

Alfalfa Seed Lupus

Other studies further support the notion that SLE is related to B_6 antimetabolites. Some monkeys fed a diet containing 40 percent oven-dried alfalfa sprouts developed a syndrome resembling human SLE. (This amount is obviously far more than any human diet would include.) In another experiment, three monkeys that were fed large amounts of alfalfa sprouts or seeds developed lupus, but the syndrome had disappeared when they resumed eating their normal monkey chow. When these animals were then placed on a semipurified diet containing 1 percent L-canavanine, a chemical present in alfalfa sprouts and seeds, their SLE was reactivated.[11]

Earlier studies of L-canavanine showed that this chemical is converted by the enzyme arginase into another molecule called L-canaline. This breakdown product was found by Gerald A. Rosenthal, Ph.D., to be a potent inhibitor of vitamin B_6-dependent enzymes.[12] Dr. Rosenthal's work suggested that the potentially toxic effect of huge amounts of alfalfa seeds and sprouts is due to L-canaline, and results from the powerful inhibition of vitamin B_6-dependent enzymes.

His work also demonstrated that the inhibitory effect of L-canaline could be reversed by supplying large amounts of pyridoxal phosphate (the active form of vitamin B_6). In the language of biochemistry, L-canaline is a competitive inhibitor of B_6-dependent enzymes. (See chapter 1 for a more detailed explanation of competitive inhibition.) Perhaps this alfalfa sprout-induced syndrome could also be prevented by supplementing the monkeys' diet with additional B_6.

Don't worry that you'll get SLE if you eat alfalfa sprouts. The monkeys were fed huge amounts of the stuff; almost any substance is toxic if taken in excess—even B_6.

The Mystery Deepens

The relationship among hydrazines, B_6 and lupus raises as many questions as it answers. For example, if B_6 is involved in SLE, why don't all patients with lupus have other B_6-responsive disorders, such as carpal tunnel syndome, premenstrual tension and monosodium glutamate intolerance? Why do some individuals develop lupus while others exposed to the same food and the same environment have no problems? Will vitamin B_6 supplements prevent SLE or relieve the symptoms in those who are already affected?

One reasonable (though hypothetical) explanation might be that a person exposed to a vitamin B_6 antagonist will not necessarily exhibit all the symptoms of B_6 deficiency. Since B_6 is a cofactor in a host of biochemical reactions performed by more than 50 different enzymes, it's possible that an antagonist would inhibit some B_6-dependent enzymes more than others. The symptoms that developed would depend on which enzymes were inhibited the most. And, since enzyme structures may differ from one person to the next, they may also differ in their capacity to hold onto the vitamin B_6 cofactor or in their ability to ward off a B_6 antagonist. Some people could develop symptoms due to an impairment of one specific enzyme, while the rest of the B_6-related machinery would continue to function normally. SLE might be likely to occur in someone whose PGE1-synthesizing enzyme (delta-6-desaturase) is unusually susceptible to B_6 antagonists.

Whether vitamin B_6 supplements will prove effective for prevention or treatment of SLE can be answered only by further research. It is encouraging that pyridoxal phosphate can reverse the antimetabolic effect of L-canaline. Unfortunately, many of the B_6 antagonists discussed in this book are noncompetitive inhibitors of B_6 (see chapter 1). In other words, even massive supplementation with B_6 may only partly reverse the damage caused by these chemicals.

In addition to B_6 supplements, successful prevention and treatment of SLE may therefore require a thorough purge of all B_6 antagonists. We would have to get rid of fried, artificially colored and overprocessed foods. We'd have to locate a source of produce that has been grown without herbicides, ripening agents or sprout inhibitors. We'd avoid using oral contraceptives or other drugs known to deplete vitamin B_6, and we'd abstain from smoking cigarettes. In addition, Dr. Rosenthal's data suggest that patients with lupus might be sensitive to alfalfa sprouts.

Hope for a Nontoxic Treatment

The only way we will ever know whether we can wipe out SLE with vitamin B_6 supplements and environmental control is to try them. If it turns out that we can't, no one will have been harmed. If patients with SLE do improve, then we'll have a new, nontoxic therapy at our disposal. Perhaps insurance companies might even begin to reimburse the additional cost of organically grown food. Aside from being a serious illness from a medical standpoint, SLE is also expensive. It is not unusual for patients with SLE to cost their insurance companies tens of thousands of dollars in hospital bills, medications and disability payments. In the long run, unprocessed, chemical-free food may be cheaper medicine than what we now have to offer.

The idea that this treatment approach might work is more than just abstract biochemical theory and wishful thinking. At least one physician has found dietary therapy of autoimmune disorders to be quite helpful. Max Gerson, M.D., a controversial physician practicing in New York several decades ago, devised a nutritional therapy that apparently helped a number of patients with SLE and other autoimmune diseases. Dr. Gerson's diet was free from pesticides, food additives and animal protein. He also prescribed various nutritional supplements. Although Dr. Gerson's dietary therapy was never accepted by the medical establishment, many patients swear that the Gerson diet has helped them. If Dr. Gerson's diet is indeed valuable in some cases of SLE, then some of its benefits may be due to elimination of vitamin B_6 antagonists from the diet.

Jonathan Wright, M.D., of Kent, Washington, has found vitamin B_6 to be quite helpful for one patient suffering from SLE.[13] Because of its theoretical benefit in autoimmune diseases, Dr. Wright has prescribed 200 to 300 milligrams of B_6 three times a day for several lupus patients (an amount to be taken only under a doctor's care). One of his patients notices definite improvement in her symptoms as long as she takes her B_6. However, if she forgets to take this vitamin, even for just a day or two, she begins to feel considerably worse.

Of course, a single case does not constitute proof. In fact, other patients with lupus have seen no apparent reduction in symptoms while taking B_6. Obviously, we still have a great deal to learn about lupus. As research clarifies the relationship between B_6 antagonists and autoimmune diseases, we may find that these chemicals play a causal role in SLE. Perhaps this discovery will not only help conquer SLE but will bring us to our senses about the way we are polluting the earth.

Chapter
Kidney
Stones 11

Kidney stones are an important medical problem in developed countries. An estimated 1 of every 15 men (and probably half as many women) in the United States has calcium oxalate kidney stones, and the number of stones has nearly doubled in the past 20 years. People who have had one stone have a 50-50 chance of developing another one, and up to age 50, they have an 8 to 10 percent chance of a recurrence in any given year.[1] As of 1978, the annual cost of medical treatment for this common urinary tract disorder was about $50 million. As we shall see, deficiencies of vitamin B_6 and magnesium appear to play a role in the development of stones.

Kidney stones vary in size from tiny pellets to large stones. They are often asymptomatic; that is, you may have one without being aware of it. Stones may pass quietly on their own, causing little difficulty except mild abdominal discomfort, but the passage of a stone can also be excruciatingly painful. In a typical attack, severe cramping pain starts in your side or your back and usually travels to your inner thigh or genitals.

Severe pain is not the only problem kidney stones may cause. If they are large enough, or if they get caught in the wrong place, the stones may block the flow of urine, causing recurrent urinary tract infections or kidney swelling. If the obstruction persists, it could lead to irreversible kidney damage. As many as one in every three people with kidney stones in the upper urinary tract eventually loses a kidney.

In the United States, about 80 to 90 percent of kidney stones contain calcium. In half these stones, the calcium is combined with oxalate, a molecule found in food and produced in the body. As you might expect, these stones are called calcium oxalate stones. Most other calcium stones also contain phosphate.

A stone begins to form when calcium oxalate dissolved in the urine precipitates (falls out of solution) and crystallizes. Once a crystal has formed, it attracts more and more calcium oxalate molecules and the crystal grows. Some stones make their way out through the urinary stream before they become too large. Others, unable to pass, continue to grow to the point where they cause trouble.

Once kidney stones have formed, all a doctor can do is try to minimize the damage, so it's important that we try to prevent the stones from occurring in the first place.

Preventive Treatments

The strategy for preventing stones can be stated quite simply: Keep the calcium and oxalate dissolved in the urine. This sounds easy, but it can get rather complicated, since urine is an extremely complex fluid. Urine contains many substances that interact in ways that are not fully understood. One group of these substances is the inhibitors, so called because they somehow prevent calcium oxalate crystals from forming. Magnesium, citrate and glutamate, three molecules normally found in the blood and urine, appear to inhibit stone formation. How they do this is unclear, but if we knew a way to increase the concentration of these molecules in the urine, we could probably keep stones from forming. Unfortunately, we don't yet have a reliable way of getting more citrate or glutamate into the urine. If you were to ingest citrate (citric acid) or glutamate (glutamic acid), most of it would be converted into other compounds before it reached the urine. Fortunately, it's not difficult to increase the urinary concentration of magnesium. You simply eat magnesium-rich foods, like green leafy vegetables or whole grains, or take magnesium supplements. Magnesium salts have been used to prevent kidney stones as long ago as the seventeenth century, but only in the past 15 years have researchers shown that the treatment actually works. In a 1982 study,[2] 55 patients with recurrent kidney stones were treated daily with 500 milligrams of magnesium. Before starting treatment, these patients were developing an average of 0.8 stones per person each year. After taking magnesium supplements for up to four years, the number of new stones decreased by 90 percent.

The concentration of solutes (dissolved molecules) in the urine is another factor that affects crystal formation. Small amounts of calcium and oxalate can easily remain dissolved without precipitating, but the greater the concentration of these molecules in the urine, the more likely they will precipitate and crystallize. Many recurrent kidney stone formers excrete abnormally large amounts of calcium, oxalate or both in their urine, so doctors have looked for ways to lower the urinary concentration of these molecules. The simplest and most effective method is to increase urine volume by drinking more water, diluting these particles and making it more difficult for crystals to form. Everyone who has had a kidney stone should be sure to drink adequate amounts of liquid. Many doctors recommend at least two and a half quarts daily.

Approximately 50 percent of people with recurrent kidney stones have hypercalciuria—an abnormally high concentration of calcium in their urine. For many years, doctors have advised stone formers to reduce their dietary calcium by eliminating dairy products. It now appears that lowering calcium intake is not a good idea, however. In the first place, eating less calcium often fails to decrease the amount of this mineral in the urine. Stone formers somehow compensate for dietary changes by drawing additional calcium from their bones, so reducing dietary calcium could lead to premature thinning of the bones. In addition, the amount of calcium in the urine is not as important as doctors had once thought. Except in cases where calcium levels are extremely high, there is little relationship between urinary calcium and the risk of stone formation.[3] For those in whom urinary calcium is important, the concentration can often be reduced by increasing dietary fiber[4] and reducing consumption of sugar,[5] meat[6] and salt.[1]

While the level of urinary calcium does not appear to be particularly important, the same cannot be said for oxalate. There is a strong relationship between oxalate excretion and stone disease.[3] Mild hyperoxaluria (increased urinary oxalate) is more common than hypercalciuria in stone formers. Although urinary oxalate is only slightly elevated in most of these people, even small increases can affect stone formation, so it's more important to lower urinary oxalate than to worry about calcium.

One common strategy for reducing urinary oxalate excretion is to avoid foods high in oxalate, such as spinach, chard, rhubarb, parsley, beet tops, tea, cola and cocoa. Although this approach is sometimes effective, this molecule is also manufactured by the body. Oxalate can be produced from two different compounds: ascorbic acid (vitamin C) and glyoxylate. Ascorbic acid is derived from food and from vitamin C supplements. Glyoxylate is a breakdown product of certain amino acids, including glycine and serine.

Vitamin C—Cause or Cure?

There has been a good deal of controversy about whether vitamin C causes kidney stones. Since this vitamin can be converted to oxalate, taking large amounts could theoretically cause a stone to develop—an especially frightening possibility, since millions of Americans take vitamin C supplements. One study showed that you can take up to 4 grams (4,000 milligrams) of vitamin C a day without producing a statistically significant increase in urinary oxalate.[7] Larger doses, say, 8 grams a day, can double urinary oxalate excretion, but even in these large amounts, vitamin C doesn't cause stones, according to nutrition-oriented doctors who have prescribed large doses of C for many years.[7] In fact, there are several ways in which vitamin C might help *prevent* stones. First, increasing the urinary concentration of vitamin C acidifies the urine, reducing calcium oxalate's tendency to precipitate. Second, vitamin C in the urine binds calcium ions, leaving less calcium available to combine with oxalate. Third, vitamin C acts as a mild diuretic,[7] and by increasing the urine flow, it dilutes the calcium and oxalate, making crystal formation less likely.

Although we needn't worry that vitamin C supplements will cause kidney stones, there are a few rare instances when vitamin C supplements have made urinary oxalate skyrocket. The tendency to react adversely to vitamin C is probably inherited. People who have had a kidney stone or who have a relative that has had stones should consult a doctor before taking vitamin C supplements. Fortunately, even these "high risk" individuals can often take vitamin C supplements safely with the help of a nutrition-oriented physician and vitamin B_6 supplements.

How B_6 Works

Vitamin B_6 may be necessary to prevent the body from producing too much oxalate. This was first pointed out in 1959 when Stanley

Gershoff, Ph.D., and co-workers found that cats fed a diet deficient in B_6 excreted unusually large amounts of oxalate in their urine, and developed calcium oxalate nephrocalcinosis (calcification of the kidney).[8]

Scientists believe that B_6 may affect oxalate production through its role in metabolism of glyoxylate. When B_6 levels are normal, more glyoxylate will be converted to glycine than to oxalate. When B_6 levels are low, more oxalate will be produced.[9] Dr. Gershoff wondered whether B_6 supplements would prevent stones in humans, so he and his colleague, Edwin L. Prien, Sr., M.D., decided to test B_6 together with magnesium supplements (already shown effective). Thirty-six patients who had at least four calcium oxalate stones in the previous two years were studied.[10] Each patient took a daily supplement containing 200 milligrams of magnesium oxide (equivalent to about 120 milligrams of magnesium) and 10 milligrams of vitamin B_6. After five years on this program, 30 of the 36 patients had either no recurrence of stones or a decrease in the number of recurrences. Analysis of their urine showed that their ability to maintain calcium oxalate in solution had improved.

Because of these encouraging results, Drs. Gershoff and Prien decided to repeat their study with a larger number of patents.[11] With the help of a group of urologists, they recruited 149 recurrent stone formers. Each patient took 300 milligrams of magnesium oxide (equivalent to about 180 milligrams of magnesium) and 10 milligrams of pyridoxine daily for four and one-half to six years. Before receiving this treatment, the group had formed an average of 1.3 stones per person per year. During therapy with magnesium and B_6, the average fell to 0.1 per person per year, an improvement of better than 90 percent, with no serious side effects.

These results are exciting. Here was a simple, safe and inexpensive treatment that could reduce the incidence of kidney stones by more than 90 percent!

Even though the B_6 and magnesium therapy had worked, the results of the initial study were somewhat confusing. On the average, urinary oxalate excretion hadn't changed and urinary magnesium levels had increased only slightly, so it was difficult to determine exactly why the treatment had helped. Also, there was no way to tell whether the results had been due mainly to B_6, magnesium or both.

In light of the evidence that magnesium supplements alone prevent kidney stones, we might question whether B_6 produces any additional benefit. Perhaps the results achieved by Drs. Gershoff and Prien were due to the slight increase in urinary magnesium levels that resulted from the treatment. If the B_6 supplement didn't reduce oxalate excretion, then perhaps it didn't really do any good. But notice that the people Drs. Gershoff and Prien studied had normal oxalate levels, even before they started taking B_6 supplements. Perhaps vitamin B_6 is helpful only when urinary oxalate levels are initially high.

Research to date suggests that B_6 supplements, even in low doses, do reduce oxalate levels in hyperoxaluric people. A group of doctors in India gave 10 milligrams of B_6 daily to 12 recurrent stone formers.[9] Before therapy, these patients were excreting quite a bit of oxalate in their urine. After 90 days on B_6, oxalate excretion decreased significantly. After 180 days, it decreased even further. This study showed that relatively small amounts of B_6 reduce oxalate excretion *in hyperoxaluric patients*.

Whether or not stone formers with normal oxalate levels should also take B_6 is a matter of opinion. It's true that we don't know whether magnesium's benefits will be boosted by a B_6 supplement. On the other hand, the 10-milligram dosage of B_6 is inexpensive and quite safe. There would be little to lose by including B_6 in the treatment of all calcium oxalate stone formers. While we do not yet have a clear rationale for using this vitamin in stone formers with normal oxalate levels, it would be dangerous to deviate from an effective treatment regimen merely because we don't think a certain portion of that treatment is necessary.

As with other effective remedies, Drs. Gershoff and Prien may have discovered the right therapy for the wrong reasons. Conceivably, B_6 might prevent kidney stones in a way that is totally unrelated to oxalate. As I mentioned earlier, glutamate is one of the compounds in urine that inhibits calcium oxalate crystallization.[12] People who suffer from kidney stones frequently have little or no glutamate in their their urine,[13] which probably contributes to the development of stones. Israeli researchers have recently discovered that low glutamate levels in the urine may be related to an enzyme deficiency. This enzyme, called glutamic oxalacetic transaminase (GOT), manufactures glutamic acid from another amino acid, aspartic acid. If this enzyme isn't working normally, then the amount of glutamic acid in the urine might be reduced. The Israeli researchers measured the urinary level of GOT in stone formers and found it was below normal. They also found abnormally low levels of another enzyme, glutamic pyruvic transaminase (GPT), which produces glutamic acid from alanine.[12,14] When GOT was mixed with the urine of stone formers, it reduced the tendency of calcium oxalate to precipitate.[14] If there were some way to correct this enzyme deficiency in the urine of stone formers, we might be able to prevent further stones from forming.

Vitamin B_6 might fit into this rather complicated scheme through its effect on GOT and GPT. B_6 is the cofactor for these enzymes; a deficiency of this vitamin would therefore reduce GOT and GPT activity. Conversely, B_6 supplements might increase the activity of these enzymes or stimulate the body to produce more of them.

All this discussion about glutamate, urinary enzymes and vitamin B_6 is still hypothetical. Further research may or may not show that B_6 supplements can increase urinary glutamate or enzyme levels. The point is that B_6 could affect stone formation in a number of different ways. For this reason, it would be unwise to neglect the vitamin just because a stone former might have a normal oxalate level.

Some Special Cases

Under certain circumstances, B_6 can dramatically affect oxalate metabolism. The first is a rare genetic disorder called primary oxalosis. Its victims excrete large amounts of oxalate and develop frequent and severe kidney stones. In some cases they die of kidney failure. Studies have shown that large doses of B_6 will decrease oxalate production in some people with primary oxalosis. In one report,[15] two patients were treated with 1,000 milligrams of B_6 a day. Urinary oxalate levels decreased in these individuals by 60 and 70 percent, respectively, and the passage of stones ceased. One of these patients had chronic renal (kidney) failure as a result of the continued damage from calcium oxalate crystals. Normally, chronic renal failure does not improve; it either stays the same or gets worse. But after 20 months of B_6 therapy, this patient's kidney function did improve. Other investigators have used smaller doses of B_6 for primary oxalosis. Although good results were achieved in some cases, others failed to improve. It is possible that some of these patients would have responded to larger amounts of B_6.

B_6 therapy has also produced definite benefits in patients with chronic renal failure who are receiving dialysis treatments. Oxalate tends to accumulate in patients with severe kidney failure and probably accounts for the calcium oxalate deposits that develop throughout their bodies, causing numerous complications. Researchers treated eight chronic renal failure patients with large doses of vitamin B_6.[16] Some received 600 milligrams daily by mouth; others were given an intravenous injection (600 milligrams) after each dialysis treatment. After four weeks of B_6 treatment, plasma oxalate levels declined an average of 46 percent. Of course, kidney patients must not take anything without the consent of their doctor. Vitamin B_6 may also be useful for people who excrete large amounts of oxalate when they take ascorbic acid (vitamin C). Much research suggests that taking vitamin C each day will help promote optimum health and prevent various diseases. (Levels above 1,000 milligrams of vitamin C a day should be taken only with your doctor's O.K.) In the vast majority of cases, doses of vitamin C as high as 9 grams a day won't greatly affect oxalate excretion. But abnormally high oxalate levels do occasionally occur in people who take large amounts of vitamin C. Jonathan Wright, M.D., of Kent, Washington, consulted with a patient who wanted to know whether it was safe to take 8,000 milligrams of vitamin C a day. Dr. Wright found that the patient's urinary oxalate excretion was very high when he took this much vitamin C. Normally, oxalate output is less than 40 milligrams daily, but this man was excreting 383 milligrams a day. After the patient began taking 50 milligrams of vitamin B_6 twice a day (without stopping the vitamin C), his urinary oxalate excretion fell to 57 milligrams a day.[17] If you are taking large amounts of vitamin C, it would be wise to have your 24-hour urinary oxalate excretion measured. If it is high, you might be able to reduce it by taking additional B_6.

Chapter
Arthritis and 12
Muscle Spasm

Arthritis, which literally means "inflammation of the joints," is one of the most common medical problems, affecting tens of millions of Americans. Although hundreds of millions of dollars are spent annually on its treatment, many arthritis victims continue to suffer pain, stiffness, weakness, loss of function, swelling and deformity in one or more joints of the body.

A special branch of medicine known as rheumatology deals primarily with studying and treating the more than 100 kinds of arthritis, some of which are relatively common and others rare. Although we know that infection, injury and allergic reactions cause arthritis, the cause of most cases remains unknown.

Modern drug therapy doesn't eliminate the cause of the arthritis in most cases; it merely relieves the symptoms temporarily. For some people, even the most up-to-date medications fail to provide adequate relief. Most arthritis sufferers have experimented with one or more alternative treatments. Obviously, the results of standard therapy usually leave something to be desired. The potential side effects of anti-inflammatory drugs are also a major cause of concern. The group of commonly used medications known as nonsteroidal anti-inflammatory agents (Indocin, Feldene, Motrin, Naprosyn, Tolectin and others) can cause nausea, vomiting, heartburn and peptic ulcers. Many arthritic patients taking one of these drugs have required emergency hospital-ization because of a bleeding peptic ulcer. Anti-inflammatory medica-tions have also caused swelling, headaches, ringing in the ears, jaundice or kidney damage. Aspirin, which is also used frequently for arthritis, can produce some of the same problems that the nonsteroidal drugs cause.

B_6-Responsive Arthritis

In one particular type of arthritis, these dangerous medicines are unnecessary, since vitamin B_6 therapy seems to relieve the problem. Unlike rheumatoid or osteoarthritis, this type of arthritis has no special name. Vitamin B_6-responsive arthritis most closely resembles what used to be called *rheumatism*, a term now rarely used. According to *Stedman's Medical Dictionary*, rheumatism is "an indefinite term applied to various conditions with pain or other symptoms which are of articular origin [arising from the joints] or related to other elements of the musculo-skeletal system." Now that arthritis can be classified into more than 100 types, there is less need (and less tolerance) for such a vague term. Nevertheless, people who suffer from the various muscle and joint aches that used to be called rheumatism frequently improve with vitamin B_6 therapy. I term this syndrome vitamin B_6-responsive arthritis.

John M. Ellis, M.D., a family doctor from Mount Pleasant, Texas, first discovered the value of vitamin B_6 for arthritis. In his 1973 book *Vitamin B_6: The Doctor's Report*,[1] Dr. Ellis described his experience in treating thousands of patients, many of them arthritic, with vitamin B_6. He began to recognize a pattern to the symptoms that would respond to this vitamin: swelling, numbness, tingling, reduced sense of touch in the fingers and hands, and pain in the finger joints, which impaired hand movements and weakened the grip. In more severe cases, patients suffered pain and stiffness in the shoulders and sometimes the elbows as well. Some also experienced swelling and/or pain in the knees, the muscles between the shoulders and elbows, or the arms and chest. Patients also complained of muscle spasms in the back of the legs and arches of the feet, locking of the finger joints and restless legs.

Dr. Ellis found that this entire group of symptoms would usually respond to 50 milligrams a day of vitamin B_6, when they weren't due to injury and were associated with the other symptoms of "rheumatism." (Isolated symptoms such as a swollen knee or a painful shoulder usually didn't improve with B_6 therapy.) Aside from relieving the pain and swelling, B_6 therapy helped arthritis patients whose arms would "fall asleep" at night. Many would lose five to seven pounds following B_6 treatment, apparently because the vitamin helped eliminate excess fluid. In some cases, Heberden's nodes (small bony protrusions near the fingertips) shrank and became less painful. Dr. Ellis found vitamin B_6 to be most effective in middle-aged women with Heberden's nodes and arthritis of the interphalangeal joints (the middle group of knuckles), a syndrome known as "menopausal arthritis."

Relief often began after several days and progressed as the B_6 treatment continued. The vitamin usually relieved elbow pain and improved finger flexion in about six weeks. Nocturnal arm paralysis, muscle cramps, weak grip, and tactile sensation usually improved within two weeks.

Despite these impressive results, Dr. Ellis's important discoveries were not given much attention by the orthodox medical community. None of his patients had been given a placebo, so it was conceivable that the improvements were purely psychological. Of course, given the dangers of modern anti-inflammatory drugs, physicians should have jumped at the chance to try a nontoxic alternative. Even though there was no obvious reason to believe that vitamin B_6 was related to arthritis, the dramatic results spoke for themselves.

Recognizing the importance of his work, Dr. Ellis teamed up with a group of researchers to discover a biochemical rationale for his B_6 treatment. Along with Karl Folkers, Ph.D., and others, Dr. Ellis studied 11 patients suffering from a group of symptoms that had typically responded to vitamin B_6.

Using EGOT measurements (described in chapter 1), they determined that these patients were deficient in vitamin B_6.[2] After daily treatment with 300 milligrams of B_6, the laboratory results gradually normalized and the symptoms disappeared or improved. It took a rather long time for the vitamin deficiency to be corrected, even with this large daily dose. After 6 weeks, the laboratory abnormalities and the clinical symptoms had only partly improved. By 11 weeks, however, both the vitamin B_6 deficiency and most of the symptoms had disappeared. In general, the clinical and laboratory improvements appeared to coincide, suggesting that B_6 deficiency was indeed the cause of the symptoms.

In my own practice, I've found this simple treatment quite helpful. L.G. was a typical patient. A 58-year-old woman with a five-year history of musculoskeletal symptoms, she had chronic "soreness" in her arms, neck and shoulders, and an aching, burning sensation in the muscles of her arms. She complained of pains around the breastbone that the local arthritis clinic had diagnosed as costochondritis (inflammation of the cartilage between the ribs and sternum). In addition, she had carpal tunnel syndrome (see chapter 13). L.G. had tried various medications, including Indocin, Clinoril, Naprosyn and Feldene, but had been forced to discontinue them because each produced intolerable abdominal pain.

This patient suspected that eating dairy products or citrus fruits made her symptoms worse. Accordingly, I asked her to stop eating these foods. I also prescribed vitamin B_6, 100 milligrams twice a day, backed up by a B-complex tablet containing 50 milligrams of each of the B vitamins. Since B_6 and magnesium work as a team, I also prescribed a tablet containing 150 milligrams of magnesium and 375 milligrams of calcium. For general support, L.G. also took a multiple vitamin and mineral tablet. After about three weeks, her carpal tunnel syndrome and costochondritis were no longer bothering her. The pains in her shoulders, neck and arms were considerably better, though not entirely gone. After five months, she continues to do well. Whenever she eats an excess of citrus or dairy products, her neck and shoulders hurt more, but not as much as before she had started taking vitamins. Her costochondritis, carpal tunnel syndrome and aching muscles are no longer a problem, even when she eats her offending foods. She is currently taking 100 milligrams of B_6 a day, which seems to work as well as the larger dose.

The case of L.G. demonstrates that several different factors may contribute to arthritis in the same individual. It seemed that her symptoms were related both to food allergy and to the need for additional vitamins. We will probably never know the exact contribution vitamin B_6 has made to L.G.'s improvement, because she is being treated with more than just B_6 supplements. What's important, however, is that L.G. and many other patients with the symptoms described by Dr. Ellis have improved with a nutritional program that includes vitamin B_6 in doses of 50 to 300 milligrams a day. (No one should exceed 50 milligrams a day without a physician's supervision.) If we are to prove once and for all that there is such a thing as B_6-responsive arthritis, we must motivate one of the large research centers to perform a double-blind trial. Such a study would be neither expensive nor technically difficult to perform. While we are waiting to discover whether B_6 is really just a placebo, we can be content in the knowledge that, for certain people, B_6 is at least as good a placebo as the expensive and dangerous nonsteroidal anti-inflammatory drugs.

Relieving Muscle Spasm

Because magnesium is known to help prevent muscle spasm[3] and vitamin B_6 supports the biochemical actions of magnesium, I have occasionally tried intravenous injections of these two nutrients for patients suffering from acute or chronic muscle spasms. Most of these patients were already taking these nutrients by mouth without benefit. Of about a dozen patients given B_6 and magnesium injections, more than half responded quite dramatically. Unfortunately, the effects of the injection don't last long; a few hours to a few days is the average. Still, this treatment appears to be worthwhile for acute muscle spasms or for flare-ups of a chronic problem.

Mrs. R., a 57-year-old woman, came to my office in May of 1983. She complained that over the past three years she had been having "terrible spasms" in her hands. These episodes would usually occur about twice a month. The first thing she noticed during these attacks was that her hands had fallen asleep. A few seconds later, as she described it, "my fingers draw up like a claw, and I have the most excruciating cramps imaginable in the front of my wrists and over the back of my hands." Sometimes her toes, feet and ankles or knees would spasm. "My toes spread out, and my feet hurt so badly that I am unable to walk on them," she told me. The severe cramping pains would usually subside after about 30 minutes, but she would continue to feel uncomfortable for much longer. "For as long as three or four days after one of these episodes, I feel as if someone is stepping on my hands," she complained.

Mrs. R. had seen a rheumatologist, who was unable to determine the cause of her troublesome symptoms. He had prescribed various medications for her, including Indocin, Clinoril, Motrin and Vasodilan. None of these drugs had helped, although Butazolidan Alka (a powerful anti-inflammatory compound) had provided some relief. She took it whenever her symptoms became intolerable.

Mrs. R. had a strong craving for sweets, but she was aware that overdoing it on the sugar would frequently trigger one of her attacks. Her glucose metabolism problem was confirmed when her blood sugar fell to 45 milligrams percent and she passed out during a six-hour glucose tolerance test. (The normal blood sugar level is 60 to 110 milligrams percent.) Mrs. R. found that she would have less-frequent and less-severe spasms if she avoided refined sugar, but she still considered these attacks a serious problem when she consulted me.

With the exception of a moderately elevated sedimentation rate, common in arthritics and indicating the presence of inflammation somewhere in her body, all other laboratory tests her rheumatologist and I performed were normal. I asked Mrs. R. to do her best to avoid refined sugar, caffeine and alcohol, and to eat small, frequent meals. I also wrote a prescription for a multiple vitamin and mineral formula, additional calcium, magnesium, vitamin B complex, and vitamins E and C. This program was designed to help improve her glucose metabolism and prevent her severe cramps from recurring.

Mrs. R. came in one week later on an "emergency visit." She was experiencing the early symptoms of one of her attacks. The fingers on her right hand looked like the claw that she had previously described, and the pain in her hand was beginning to build. I drew 150 milligrams of pyridoxine and 600 milligrams of magnesium chloride into a syringe and slowly injected it intravenously. Before the injection had even been completed, Mrs. R. expressed amazement that her spasm had disappeared. Her fingers were no longer clenched, and she reported no further pain.

Since Mrs. R. has been eating less sugar and refined carbohydrates and taking her vitamins, her muscle cramping has subsided. When her hands did act up on several occasions, another injection of B_6 and magnesium relieved her symptoms within seconds.

This combination injection has also been helpful for a 63-year-old woman suffering from chronic muscle spasms in her upper back, neck and throat. Mrs. M. had a long history of degenerative arthritis (osteoarthritis) of the cervical spine. Previous X rays had shown that a degenerating disc in her neck was putting pressure on one of her cervical nerves. Apparently she was caught in a vicious cycle. The pain resulting from compression of the nerve would cause certain muscles in her neck and shoulders to tighten up. This would put additional pressure on the nerve, which would in turn make the muscle spasm worse. Often the pain and stiffness would become so severe that she could barely turn her neck. Mrs. M. also noticed a feeling like a lump in her throat during her most severe muscle spasms. Although anti-inflammatory medications helped a little, they didn't help enough. She had been advised by a neurosurgeon that the only chance for lasting improvement was to correct the nerve compression surgically.

In May of 1983, when her spasms were bothering her more than usual, I gave Mrs. M. an intravenous injection of vitamin B_6 (200 milligrams) and magnesium chloride (600 milligrams). Immediately after the two-minute injection, she was amazed that the pain in her back and the lump in her throat had disappeared. Although she could barely move her neck before the injection, she now had almost full range of motion in all directions without pain. Unfortunately, the effect of the injection lasted only about 24 hours. Subsequent injections during periods of acute pain would last anywhere from six hours to three days. Each time, however, the results were immediate. On one occasion I gave Mrs. M. a three-hour intravenous drip of vitamin B_6 (400 milligrams), magnesium chloride (4,000 milligrams), vitamin-B-complex injectable (1 cc), and vitamin C (2,500 milligrams). She remained free of all symptoms for nine days after this injection. Her chiropractor reports that her spine is considerably easier to manipulate after she receives one of her injections.

Mrs. M. now requests B_6 and magnesium injections only during severe flare-ups. The injections haven't cured her problems, but they allow her to make it through her worst times with considerably less discomfort. Although she takes vitamin B_6 and magnesium by mouth, they don't appear to help her spasms. Some of the improvements Mrs. M. feels could be a placebo effect; patients often experience symptom relief merely because they have been given an injection. I've seen this same immediate relief in several other patients, however, even though they were told the benefits might not be felt until the next day, so it's unlikely that the improvement is due entirely to a placebo effect.

Obviously, intravenous injections of anything, including vitamins and minerals, should not be taken lightly. Although adverse reactions to B_6 or low-dose magnesium injections are extremely rare, they can occur (especially if one is allergic to the preservative in the injection solution). Intravenous B_6 and magnesium is not a cure for muscle spasm, but my brief experience with a dozen or so patients suggests it's sometimes a useful alternative to short-term therapy with standard muscle relaxants or anti-inflammatory drugs. I have not yet figured out which of these nutrients is more important for relieving muscle spasm. In the few cases where they were tried individually, the combination appeared to work better than either magnesium or B_6 alone. Further research will give us a better idea of when these injections are most likely to be beneficial.

Medical nutritionists also recommend other nutritional supplements for arthritis—usually niacinamide, vitamin E, zinc and copper. Some patients also notice definite relief when they eliminate from their diet foods to which they're allergic. Nutritional therapy is often quite effective for arthritis, and many people who have tried this approach have been able to throw away their drugs and live less-painful and more-active lives.

Chapter
Carpal 13
Tunnel
Syndrome

The median nerve, a major nerve for sensory and motor function in the hand and wrist, passes through the carpal tunnel, located at the wrist, just above the palm of the hand. Carpal tunnel syndrome arises when the median nerve becomes compressed. Its symptoms include burning, tingling and either increased or decreased sensation in the thumb, the first two fingers and the adjacent half of the ring finger. The syndrome can pose major difficulties for carpenters, tailors, housewives or other people who have to use their hands frequently.

Since swelling of tissues around the median nerve often causes these symptoms, the usual treatment is anti-inflammatory medication or cortisone injections to reduce the swelling. When these drugs fail to work, hand surgery is often recommended to release some of the pressure on the median nerve. But even surgery doesn't always work, and some people develop the symptoms again months or years after the operation.

Carpal tunnel syndrome has become much more common since George Phalen, M.D., first described it at the 99th annual meeting of the American Medical Association in 1950. At that time, very few of the doctors present had ever heard of it; today every family doctor frequently sees median nerve compression. During the same three decades, a number of vitamin B_6 antimetabolites entered our environment. The syndrome also occurs fairly frequently in women who are either pregnant or taking birth control pills,[1] both of which promote B_6 deficiency. These connections constitute circumstantial evidence that B_6 is related to median nerve compression.

John M. Ellis, M.D., Karl Folkers, Ph.D., and their colleagues at the University of Texas, Austin, have treated many hundreds of patients suffering from carpal tunnel syndrome. They found that vitamin B_6, usually in daily doses of 50 milligrams, relieved the symptoms nearly every time. Sometimes patients responded rapidly; in other cases, they took 6 or even 12 weeks to improve. Dr. Ellis also observed that these patients frequently had swollen hands and fingers, and that vitamin B_6 usually relieved this as well.

When Dr. Ellis reported his findings in his 1973 book,[2] medical nutritionists were excited. Dr. Ellis had discovered a safe and effective treatment for a common problem that had previously been treatable only with drugs and surgery. It soon became clear to nearly every doctor who tried it that B_6 indeed worked most of the time. Of course, if the case was so advanced that irreversible tissue damage had occurred, or if the nerve compression was caused by a prior fracture or the structural deformities of rheumatoid arthritis, the vitamin was unlikely to help. But in the great majority of cases, vitamin B_6 effectively eliminated the symptoms.

The orthodox medical community showed little interest in Dr. Ellis's work. Because the symptoms of carpal tunnel syndrome can come and go unpredictably, most doctors passed off the cures with vitamin B_6 as "spontaneous remissions." It didn't seem to matter to the skeptics that, in hundreds of cases, the symptoms didn't come back unless the patient stopped taking the vitamin. Nor did it seem to matter that any doctor could easily verify or refute Dr. Ellis's claims merely by trying B_6 on a few patients. As usual, the burden of proof rested on the shoulders of those promoting the new treatment, even though it was safer, less expensive, and apparently more effective than the alternatives available at that time.

Dr. Ellis and his colleagues have now published enough data to convince all but the closed-minded that vitamin B_6 is the treatment of choice for most cases of carpal tunnel syndrome. Even Dr. Phalen, who pioneered the surgical treatment for this syndrome, agrees that B_6 holds great promise.[3] It should not be long before all physicians are prescribing vitamin B_6 for the carpal tunnel syndrome.

Experimental Evidence

Dr. Ellis, Dr. Folkers and others had already demonstrated that people with carpal tunnel syndrome frequently show evidence of vitamin B_6 deficiency.[4] The fact that it took about the same amount of time to correct the deficiency as it did to relieve the symptoms corroborated the theory that B_6 deficiency was the cause of the problem. To convince the medical community, Dr. Ellis and co-workers performed a double-blind study and reported their results in December, 1982.[5]

Seven patients suffering from carpal tunnel syndrome were treated with pyridoxine or a placebo, each for 12 weeks. Prior to the study, all seven patients showed biochemical evidence of vitamin B_6 deficiency. When the patients received B_6, their symptoms improved significantly. On the other hand, they showed no improvement during the placebo period. Vitamin B_6 relieved symptoms, even in people who had suffered for as long as eight years.

Dr. Ellis found that symptoms may take as long as three months to respond to B_6. Apparently, the vitamin must do more than merely activate existing B_6-dependent enzymes, a process that takes only a few days. It must also increase the total number of enzyme molecules, a process called enzyme induction.

Don't Give Up

Since the full effect of enzyme induction can take weeks or even months to be felt, the response to B_6 may be slow. It's less important to understand the biochemical explanation of how B_6 works than to appreciate the importance of not giving up too soon on B_6 therapy. A few doctors have become disillusioned with B_6 after having tried it for only a week or two. Of course, some people respond more rapidly than others. I saw one middle-aged woman improve dramatically in two days. In general, the longer someone has had the problem, the longer it takes to improve. In some people with severe and long-standing symptoms, even more than 12 weeks might be required.

If you suspect that you have carpal tunnel syndrome, please see your doctor before prescribing B_6 for yourself. Your symptoms may turn out to be due to something other than median nerve compression. For example, degenerative arthritis of the upper spine could cause pressure on certain nerves and trigger symptoms similar to carpal tunnel syndrome. Hypothyroidism or other chronic illnesses can also occasionally cause median nerve compression.

The discovery that vitamin B_6 can relieve the carpal tunnel syndrome elevated the status of this important nutrient in the eyes of certain traditional nutritionists. Finally there was a disease with well-defined symptoms that could be readily diagnosed and effectively treated with vitamin B_6 alone. Not that each nutrient must be associated with a specific deficiency disease. A vitamin or mineral could play a supportive role in a host of different ways without being the single effective treatment for a specific illness, but traditional nutritionists tend to take a nutrient less seriously if it is not a magic bullet. Take vitamin E, for example. Despite hundreds of reports attesting to its therapeutic value, E is still disparagingly referred to by the orthodoxy as "a vitamin in search of a disease." Now that a disease has been found for B_6, perhaps doctors will be more inclined to take a close look at some of its other uses.

Part V

Overcoming Common Problems

Chapter
Anemia 14

Anemia is defined as an abnormally low level of either the number or volume (hematocrit) of red blood cells, or the amount of hemoglobin in a given amount of blood. The principle function of hemoglobin and of the red cells that house this protein is to transport oxygen to the various tissues and organs of the body. Hemoglobin picks up oxygen from the lungs, carries it through the bloodstream, exchanges it for a carbon dioxide molecule somewhere in the body, and then transports the carbon dioxide back to the lungs to be exhaled. Obviously, hemoglobin is essential for the most basic metabolic reactions that support life.

The usual symptoms—if any—of mild anemia are fatigue, weakness or shortness of breath, reflecting a lack of oxygen. Severe anemia also places a strain on the heart, which must compensate for "inefficient" blood by pumping it faster than usual through the body. Occasionally, anemia is the first sign of serious illness.

Anemia can be caused by excessive bleeding, rapid destruction of red blood cells or impaired production of red cells due to nutritional deficiency. The nutrient deficiencies most frequently associated with anemia are iron, folate and vitamin B_{12}. Vitamin B_6 deficiency (or dependency) is also an important, though less common, cause of anemia, since it's the coenzyme for an enzyme called delta-aminolevulinic acid synthetase (delta-ALA-synthetase), which catalyzes an important step in hemoglobin production. Vitamin B_6 deficiency or an abnormal B_6

144

metabolism can reduce the amount of hemoglobin made by the bone marrow.

Sideroblastic Anemia

The major type of anemia that responds to vitamin B_6 is called sideroblastic anemia, a disorder that is either inherited or acquired in later life. Inherited sideroblastic anemia responds to B_6 therapy much more readily than the acquired kind.[1,2] The term *sideroblastic* refers to the buildup of iron *(sidero-)* in immature blood cells *(blasts)* that results when there is some defect in hemoglobin production. Young red cells normally collect iron, a key component of every hemoglobin molecule. If, for some reason, the cells manufacture less hemoglobin, the unused iron molecules deposit themselves in the shape of a ring around the outside of the young cell's nucleus. These iron deposits give the red cell its characteristic sideroblastic appearance.

The red blood cells of people with sideroblastic anemia are usually smaller than normal and contain less than the usual amount of hemoglobin. Although this pattern resembles iron-deficiency anemia, these two types of anemia can be distinguished by a diagnostic examination of bone marrow tissue under the microscope. The bone marrow in iron-deficiency anemia lacks ringed sideroblasts. Occasionally the red cells in B_6-deficiency anemia are abnormally large and there are no sideroblasts in the bone marrow. For this reason, doctors should always consider recommending vitamin B_6 supplements in unusual cases of anemia, regardless of what the blood and bone marrow look like under the microscope.

Hereditary sideroblastic anemia is usually partly relieved by pyridoxine in doses many times the Recommended Dietary Allowance (RDA). Smaller doses don't work in most cases.[1]

John D. Hines, M.D., and David Love, Ph.D., at Case Western Reserve University found out why pyridoxine doesn't always work. They studied vitamin B_6 metabolism in 34 people whose sideroblastic anemia had not improved with pyridoxine therapy. In 18 of these cases, the ability to convert pyridoxine to biologically active pyridoxal phosphate (PLP) was impaired. Perhaps the reason these people weren't responding to B_6 was that their bodies weren't using it properly. What if the vitamin were administered as pyridoxal phosphate? Would it correct the anemia? In order to find out, these doctors gave the 18 patients with abnormal B_6 metabolism an injection of 25 to 50 milligrams of PLP four times a day for eight to ten days. Hemoglobin levels rose significantly in 11 of the 18 patients who received this treatment.[3] Unfortunately, injectable PLP isn't yet available. PLP tablets have recently been marketed by several different vitamin companies, however. Although oral PLP is relatively expensive, and some experimental evidence suggests that it is poorly absorbed, a few medical nutritionists feel that this form of vitamin B_6 works better and at lower doses than pyridoxine.

Sideroblastic anemia also occurs in people taking isoniazid and cycloserine, drugs used to treat tuberculosis. These drugs interfere with vitamin B_6 metabolism, and B_6 therapy will often correct the anemia.[4]

Other B_6-Responsive Anemias

Vitamin B_6 therapy has also been attempted in other types of difficult-to-treat anemia. One such anemia is associated with primary myelofibrosis,[5] a disease in which the body loses its ability to make red blood cells. A group of physicians from the Netherlands treated 11 patients suffering from primary myelofibrosis with 250 milligrams of pyridoxine hydrochloride daily. Within three months, 6 of the 11 patients responded to pyridoxine with a large rise in hemoglobin (at least 3 grams per 100 milliliters) or hematocrit (at least 10 percent). Because of the severity of their anemia, these 6 patients had been receiving repeated blood transfusions. After vitamin B_6 therapy, blood transfusions were no longer necessary. Vitamin B_6 thus spared these patients the nuisance, the expense and the risk of hepatitis and other reactions that accompany blood transfusions.

Folate deficiency is probably the most common cause of anemia in women taking oral contraceptives; however, the pill also promotes B_6 deficiency, which is occasionally severe enough to trigger anemia. Only one woman with B_6-responsive anemia due to birth control pills has so far been reported in the medical literature.[6] In this case, B_6 deficiency wasn't suspected until all other causes of the anemia had been ruled out. The woman's bone marrow didn't have the typical sideroblastic pattern of B_6 deficiency, but the anemia promptly cleared up once vitamin B_6 treatment was started. Perhaps this case will lead physicians to suspect B_6 deficiency more often in women who become anemic while taking the Pill.

Vitamin B_6 appears to prevent anemia either by increasing the activity of the hemoglobin synthesizer delta-ALA-synthetase or by extending the life-span of red blood cells. Future research may point to additional roles for B_6 in preventing anemia.

The Shotgun Approach

One of the classic controversies between medical nutritionists and traditional physicians is over shotgun therapy. Nutritionists often prescribe a large number of nutrients at the same time, hoping to cover all bases. Traditional physicians decry this shotgun approach, preferring instead to find and treat a specific deficiency. This attitude is an outgrowth of drug-oriented medical practice: It would certainly not be a good idea to prescribe two potentially toxic medications if only one is needed. On the other hand, in nutrition the shotgun approach is preferable, since multiple nutrient deficiencies occur more frequently than do single deficiencies, and the function of one nutrient is often dependent on the presence of adequate amounts of others. Merely taking the single nutrient most obviously lacking may not always produce the best results. Doctors have observed that a supplement containing all of the known blood-building nutrients is frequently more effective than therapy with iron, folate or vitamin B_{12} alone.[7] A reasonable argument can therefore be made that a little bit of vitamin B_6 should be used to treat all cases of anemia.

An interesting relationship between B_6 and the amino acid tryptophan has been discovered in one person with B_6-responsive anemia. This 54-year-old man had been able to control his anemia for 11 years by taking 12.5 milligrams of pyridoxine a day, off and on. Eventually this dose of B_6 failed to correct his anemia. However, when he began taking tryptophan (250 milligrams three times a day), there was a prompt improvement.[8] Perhaps tryptophan will be helpful for other individuals with sideroblastic anemia that fails to respond to vitamin B_6 alone.

A significant percentage of people with mild anemia don't respond to the usual treatment with iron, vitamin B_{12} or folate. Some of them do better when additional nutrients, such as vitamins B_6, C and E, copper and others, are added. As we continue to learn more about how nutrients interact, the treatment of anemia will no doubt improve. Remember, anemia is occasionally a sign of serious illness, so any treatment should be undertaken only with professional medical advice.

Chapter
Alcoholism 15

There are 10 million to 15 million alcoholics and problem drinkers in the United States;[1] tens of millions of other Americans drink alcoholic beverages regularly. Most of these drinkers suffer nutritional deficiencies, since alcohol tends to displace more nutritious foods when it becomes a major part of the diet. Alcohol also damages the gastrointestinal tract, interfering with the absorption of many nutrients.

Approximately 50 percent of heavy drinkers tested show laboratory evidence of vitamin B_6 deficiency. Poor diet and faulty absorption explain only partly why B_6 deficiency is so common. Another reason is that acetaldehyde, a breakdown product of alcohol, interferes with the metabolism of pyridoxal phosphate (the active form of B_6).[2] Also, the livers of chronic alcoholics often can't convert pyridoxine from food or vitamin tablets into usable form. Although moderate consumption of alcohol does not cause severe B_6 deficiency, it may put some strain on our B_6 metabolism.

B_6 deficiency contributes to some complications of alcoholism. Chronic alcohol abusers sometimes develop vitamin B_6-deficiency anemia (sideroblastic anemia)[3] or neuropathy (a disorder of the nervous system characterized by numbness, pain, weakness and other symptoms).

A Sobering Idea

Vitamin B_6 can be used to modify the acute effects of alcohol as well as its long-term consequences. Several reports from the 1950's suggest that an intravenous injection of this vitamin will convert an acutely intoxicated person into a completely sober one in a matter of minutes. V. P. Wordsworth, M.D., reported a case in the *British Medical Journal* of a 45-year-old woman who was brought to him "singing, swearing and staggering." Three minutes after she was given 100 milligrams of vitamin B_6 intravenously, she became quiet, apologized for the trouble she had caused and stated she felt quite sober.[4] Dr. Wordsworth treated five other intoxicated people with B_6 injections and found the same results in each instance. H. Pullar-Strecker, writing in the same issue of the *British Medical Journal*, remarked that intravenous injections of high-dose multiple vitamins eliminate every symptom of intoxication.[5] In another report, doctors gave 100 milligrams of vitamin B_6 intravenously to a violent alcoholic with a suspected head injury. Eight minutes later, the man became quiet, sat up in bed and was able to give a coherent account of what had happened.[6]

Intrigued by these reports, a group of scientists in Boston decided to study the effects of vitamin B_6 on drunkenness.[7] Six chronic alcoholics volunteered to be studied. Each volunteer drank an intoxicating dose of alcohol, then received an intravenous injection of pyridoxine (either 500 or 2,000 milligrams). (You should never use B_6 in these dosages without consulting your doctor.) In some of these people, evidence of intoxication disappeared and they were able to perform normal motor tasks within 15 to 45 minutes of the injection. These sobering effects occurred even though blood alcohol levels remained well above normal.

Despite these positive results, the Boston group was unimpressed; contrary to the observations of Dr. Wordsworth and others, they concluded that the effect of pyridoxine wasn't immediately striking and obvious, and they rejected the idea that B_6 injections could rapidly sober someone up. Partly because of this study, the effect of vitamin B_6 on alcoholic intoxication was forgotten.

Unfortunately, the Boston study was interpreted more negatively than it should have been. Not only did some of the volunteers become sober more quickly than expected, but the experimental conditions didn't duplicate the conditions under which B_6 had earlier been reported effective. The alcoholics studied by the Boston group rapidly drank anywhere from two-thirds of a pint to almost a full pint of whiskey and received the B_6 injection shortly thereafter. Perhaps those who had responded to B_6 in the hospital emergency room hadn't drunk as much alcohol or hadn't been given their injection so soon after drinking. Perhaps some of the volunteers in the Boston group had such badly damaged livers that they couldn't convert pyridoxine to its active form, pyridoxal phosphate.

In any case, the exciting potential of vitamin B_6 shouldn't be disregarded solely on the basis of one dissenting opinion. The effect of vitamin B_6 on alcohol intoxication clearly needs to be looked into further.

Meningitis and DT's

The possibility that pyridoxal phosphate injections might work when pyridoxine doesn't should also be investigated, especially since there are a number of situations in which a nontoxic method of sobering someone up would be quite useful. In the hospital, doctors often prescribe sedatives to control a violent or combative alcoholic. Since alcohol is itself a sedative, the combination of alcohol and tranquilizers can lead to trouble. Also, when intoxicated people are brought to the emergency room with a fever, doctors must consider the possibility that they have meningitis. The symptoms of this serious illness include fever and abnormal behavior. If diagnosis is delayed even for an hour or two, a meningitis patient could die. In order to rule out meningitis, doctors frequently subject hospitalized alcoholics to a lumbar puncture, in which a needle is inserted through the lumbar spine and fluid is drawn from the spinal canal. This procedure can cause severe headaches and can increase the risk of bacteria being introduced into the spinal canal. If an intoxicated patient with a fever could be rapidly sobered up with vitamin B_6, he might be spared the risks of a lumbar puncture.

Vitamin B_6 could also be useful in the prevention and treatment of delirium tremens (DT's), which is characterized by tremors, fumbling movements of the hands, extreme agitation, hallucinations and seizures. Delirium tremens is a medical emergency. As many as 15 percent of cases end fatally, so people in DT's must be treated with care. Although sedatives are necessary to suppress agitation and prevent exhaustion, they can also interfere with the alcoholic's breathing. Clearly, we need to add a nontoxic remedy to the standard treatment of DT's.

In some ways the symptoms of delirium tremens resemble those of severe vitamin B_6 deficiency. Lack of B_6 can cause epileptic seizures and various psychiatric symptoms. Because these are two of the symptoms of DT's, and because alcoholics are known to be low in B_6, Edwin J. Palmer, M.D., in Roanoke, Virginia, studied the effect of B_6 in several cases of delirium tremens.[8] Dr. Palmer found that 500 to 1,000 milligrams of pyridoxine given intravenously completely relieved the physical and mental manifestations of DT's within three hours. In cases where pyridoxine was used, sedation was unnecessary. Another group of doctors was unable to confirm the results obtained by Dr. Palmer. In this second study, hospitalized chronic alcoholics treated with B_6 didn't recover any faster than others who were not given the vitamin.[9] These patients had been drinking heavily for an average of 13 years. Perhaps their livers had lost the ability to manufacture pyridoxal phosphate.

Magnesium's Role

A more likely explanation for the failure of B_6 is that severe magnesium deficiency resulting from years of alcohol abuse had impaired these patients' ability to respond to this vitamin. Since B_6 and magnesium work together as a biochemical team, when one of these nutrients is lacking, the other's action can be impaired. The vast majority of chronic alcoholics are low in magnesium. In one study, the muscle tissue concentration of magnesium was below normal in nine out of ten chronic abusers of alcohol.[10]

Magnesium deficiency itself appears to be related to DT's. Animals fed a diet low in magnesium developed symptoms that resembled delirium tremens in humans. Furthermore, when a group of alcoholics was given intramuscular injections of magnesium sulfate, their symptoms of DT's often lessened or disappeared within several days.[11]

According to the observations of various researchers, large doses of vitamin B_6 might actually produce a mild magnesium deficiency. If an alcoholic is already critically short in magnesium, the beneficial effect of a vitamin B_6 injection in delirium tremens might be counterbalanced. This might explain the failure of vitamin B_6 injections in some cases of long-standing alcoholism. If we are going to prevent or effectively treat this alcohol-withdrawal syndrome, we must be sure to use both of these important nutrients together.

Liver Damage

Vitamin B_6 may also help prevent the liver damage that results from continued drinking. Ethanol, the drinkable form of alcohol, is broken down by the body to acetaldehyde, which is toxic to liver cells and appears to be a major cause of liver malfunction in alcoholics. Shin-ichi Kakuma, M.D., and colleagues at the New Jersey Medical School performed an experiment to determine whether vitamin B_6 could prevent this toxic effect in B_6-deficient patients.[12] Dr. Kakuma studied liver cells that had been obtained by biopsy from patients suffering from alcoholic hepatitis. When he mixed these cells with acetaldehyde, he found cell damage; however, when he also added pyridoxal phosphate to the test tube, acetaldehyde was significantly less toxic to the liver cells. Dr. Kakuma also found that liver cells obtained from alcoholics who had received B_6 injections were more resistant to acetaldehyde than were the cells from people who weren't treated with B_6. The results of this work suggested that correcting vitamin B_6 deficiency might help prevent liver damage in alcohol drinkers.

Since drinking alcohol tends to promote a wide range of nutritional deficiencies, some of which appear to cause certain medical problems, all nutritional deficiencies should be corrected in heavy drinkers. The medical profession is keenly aware of the need for folate and thiamine (vitamin B_1) supplements in alcoholics. It's time that other nutrients, especially vitamin B_6 and magnesium, also be given serious consideration.

Chapter

Tooth Decay 16

Despite fluoridated water supplies and regular fluoride treatments by dentists, tooth decay is still disturbingly common. By three years of age, about 57 percent of American children have at least one cavity; by school age, more than 70 percent have some tooth decay.[1] In addition to creating enormous dental bills, this cavity epidemic adversely affects our health. Proper chewing (and therefore healthy teeth) is necessary to digest food efficiently. As a rule, our natural teeth can break down food much better than dentures can, so tooth decay, the most important cause of tooth loss, is an important cause of nutritional deficiency.

Whoever said that "nature castigates those who don't masticate" was not far from the truth. In my experience, people are less likely to suffer allergic reactions to food that has been completely broken down and digested. In general, only relatively large molecules cause allergies. If the teeth do their job, there's a better chance that food will be broken down to the point where it's no longer allergenic. On the other hand, food chewed hastily or with poorly functioning teeth can cause trouble. One young man reportedly developed an annoying case of hives every time he bolted down his food. When he ate the same food slowly, he never got hives. It didn't matter *what* he ate, only *how fast*.[2] As food allergy is becoming increasingly recognized as a common cause of physical and emotional disorders, the importance of proper chewing and healthy teeth cannot be overemphasized.

Ironically, cavities are relatively rare among societies that consume unrefined foods and have no dentists or toothpastes; yet we who receive the best that modern dental science has to offer have not been able to prevent our teeth from rotting. Like so many other modern epidemics, tooth decay appears to be a disease of civilization.

The most obvious culprit is our diet. It's now well accepted that eating too much sugar will cause tooth decay, but sugar is probably not the only villain. There is evidence that vitamin B_6 deficiency may also affect tooth decay. This isn't well known, even though most of the studies on B_6 and cavities have been around for more than 20 years. Although final proof is not yet in, there are several reasons to believe that B_6 helps protect our teeth. We know that children who chew sugarcane are resistant to cavities, even if they don't take good care of their teeth. The sucrose refined from sugarcane, on the other hand, *is* an important cause of decay. Apparently, some protective factor in sugarcane is removed during the refining process. What is this protective factor present in cane but not in refined sugar? It could be vitamin B_6. The raw cane plant overflows with B_6, containing 430 parts per million. At this concentration, a single ounce of sugarcane would provide 12 milligrams of B_6, or approximately six times the Recommended Dietary Allowance (RDA) for this vitamin.

Two Types of Bacteria

Studies showing that vitamin B_6 affects mouth bacteria suggest that this important vitamin may indeed prevent cavities. The pattern of microorganisms residing in the mouth is one of the key factors involved in forming cavities. Some bacteria manufacture acidic compounds that can dissolve calcium in the tooth enamel and lead to decay. Others are less acid-forming and therefore less likely to promote tooth decay.

Studies have shown that cavity-prone people tend to harbor different strains of bacteria in their mouth than those who are free from decay. In one study, *Lactobacillus* (abbreviated *L.*) counts were measured in the saliva of a group of men drafted into the navy. Men with high *L. acidophilus* counts had numerous cavities; those with high *L. casei* counts had far fewer.[3] *L. acidophilus* is an acid-producing (and therefore cavity-promoting) strain of *Lactobacillus*, whereas *L. casei* is not. If we could somehow discourage the acid formers from setting up shop inside our mouths, we might be able to prevent tooth decay.

There is evidence that B_6 influences the type of bacteria present in the mouth. Some organisms require external supplies of this vitamin for growth and maintenance, while others can manufacture their own. If there is a B_6 deficiency in the environment, the organisms that require it won't survive. On the other hand, with adequate supplies of the vitamin, B_6-dependent organisms usually flourish and dominate other bacteria.

One of the bacteria that requires B_6 is *L. casei*, the same organism associated with a low incidence of cavities. Since B_6 doesn't support the growth of acid-forming bacteria in the mouth,[4] B_6 supplements might prevent cavities.

Most of the work on B_6-dependent bacteria has been done in the test tube, so we should be careful not to draw unwarranted conclusions about real-life situations. On the other hand, there is reason to believe that vitamin B_6 does affect bacterial populations in human beings. In the 1950's some infants fed an infant formula later found to be low in B_6 developed convulsions. When the problem was discovered, the infants were switched to another product containing more B_6. When the formula was switched, it caused a marked change in the infants' intestinal flora. There was a substantial increase in the population of *L. bifidus*, a non-acid-producing organism.[5] Of course, the mouth is the first portion of the gastrointestinal tract, and it's likely that B_6 could also produce favorable changes there.

Several decades ago, Lyon P. Strean, Ph.D., D.D.S., and colleagues tested this possibility in animals. They fed a group of hamsters a cariogenic (cavity-producing) diet.[6] Half the animals were given 50 micrograms of vitamin B_6 per 100 grams of food, an amount just sufficient for normal maintenance. The other half received 20 times as much of the vitamin. In the "normal-B_6" group, 26 percent of the tooth structure was destroyed by the diet. In those given the high-B_6 diet, only 4.2 percent of the tooth structure was lost.

Because of his animal findings, Dr. Strean decided to test vitamin B_6 in humans.[7] He recruited 28 children aged 10 to 15 and divided them into two groups. One group was given lozenges containing 3 milligrams of pyridoxine. The others were given placebo lozenges containing the same ingredients except for B_6. Each child was instructed to take three lozenges a day, one after each meal. The bottles were coded, so the children didn't know whether they were receiving B_6 or a placebo. To measure the degree of tooth decay, Dr. Strean used a standard scale known as the DMF rating. The higher the DMF rating, the more tooth decay the children had.

Children receiving the B_6 lozenges had a total score of 118 at the beginning and 170 at the end of the experiment, an increase of 52 points. Children who were given the placebo went from 109 to 196, an increase of 87 points. The vitamin supplements prevented about 40 percent of the increase in DMF ratings, a statistically significant effect.

Abram Cohen, D.D.S., and Carl Rubin, D.D.S., studied 345 children between the ages of 11 and 14.[8] They determined a DMF rating for each child beforehand. Half the children were given B_6 lozenges similar to the ones used by Dr. Strean, supplying 3 milligrams of pyridoxine. The rest of the children received placebo lozenges. To correct for any possible psychological effect on the development of cavities, the study was double-blind. Neither the dentists nor the children knew which lozenges contained the vitamin. The lozenges were taken three times a day after meals for eight months. When the study was completed, children receiving the placebo had a 26 percent greater increase in DMF ratings than those treated with B_6. Again, the B_6 group had developed fewer cavities than those receiving the placebo. This time the difference barely missed statistical significance ($p = .06$; a 6 percent probability that the results were due to chance alone), so some scientists may be inclined to ignore these results. However, if a larger number of children had been tested, perhaps the 26 percent improvement would have been statistically significant.

The work of Drs. Strean and Cohen strongly suggests that vitamin B_6 lozenges help prevent cavities in children. These findings are especially important, since the children were living in a flouridated area, so B_6 may have a protective effect above and beyond fluoride.

Some people question the safety of fluoridated water and fluoride treatment of teeth. The decision whether or not to use fluoride is, of course, an individual one (assuming that you have a way to avoid the public water supply). I am *not* recommending B_6 as a replacement for fluoride: The protective effect of B_6 is apparently in the range of only 25 to 40 percent, and most dentists will tell you that fluoride treatments and fluoridated water work a lot better than that. Using fluoride is still the most effective way to prevent cavities in children who eat typical American food. For those who decide to shun fluoride, it's reassuring that B_6 may help reduce cavities.

Decay Prevention in Pregnancy

Robert W. Hillman, M.D., Philip G. Cabaud, M.D., and Roger A. Schenone, D.D.S., performed an experiment with pregnant women[9] similar to Dr. Strean's experiment with children. Women often get cavities during or shortly after pregnancy and are often deficient in vitamin B_6 then. Could this deficiency cause the cavities? Dr. Hillman divided 540 pregnant women living in a nonfluoridated area into three groups. The first group (the controls) was given a multivitamin containing no B_6 and a supply of placebo lozenges (to be taken three times daily). Group II received a multivitamin with 20 milligrams of B_6 in it, plus three placebo lozenges. The third group was given the vitamin formula without B_6, as well as three lozenges, each containing 6.67 milligrams of B_6 (a total of 20 milligrams). Dr. Hillman was interested in finding out whether keeping B_6 in the mouth longer (with a lozenge) would be more effective than swallowing the vitamin in a capsule.

The women who received no B_6 had an average increase in DMF rating of 1.42 per person. Those who took B_6 in capsule form had an average increase of 1.22. The increase in tooth decay was 11 percent less than that of women in the placebo group (not statistically significant). The results with B_6 lozenges, however, were more pronounced. The average increase in DMF ratings among those taking the lozenges was only 0.89, or 37 percent less than the placebo group. This difference *was* statistically significant. The percentage of women showing no increase in DMF ratings was 33 for placebo, 43 for B_6 tablets and 54 for B_6 lozenges. This study demonstrated that B_6 lozenges help protect against the development of cavities in pregnant women. The 37 percent protection was similar to the findings in the studies on children. Why did the lozenges work better than the vitamin capsules? The most obvious explanation is that B_6 works primarily by changing the bacterial content of the mouth. The longer the vitamin stays in the mouth, the greater its benefits.

Most of this research was conducted more than 20 years ago and has since been forgotten. However, tooth decay remains a major public health problem despite the benefits of fluoride. So far, the evidence suggests that vitamin B_6 lozenges could play an important role in the battle against cavities. This work needs to be revived, and the effect of B_6 on the teeth must be studied more widely. If 9 milligrams a day in lozenge form gave a 25 to 40 percent benefit, then perhaps 20 or 30 milligrams a day might be even more effective. (Studies have shown that a B_6 concentration of 50 parts per million is optimal to support the growth of helpful mouth bacteria.)[4] Perhaps we will discover that larger amounts of B_6 work as well as fluoride. If so, the question of fluoride toxicity will become moot for those who use B_6. There is little chance that 20 or 30 milligrams of B_6 daily would be toxic, especially in older children, but the lozenge must be buffered properly: Vitamin B_6 supplements are usually made of pyridoxine hydrochloride, an acidic compound that could erode dental enamel with continual contact.

B_6 may protect the teeth in other ways unrelated to bacteria. Teeth are living tissues that extract nutrients from the blood and give off waste products. Like other tissues, teeth are susceptible to the effects of malnutrition. Conceivably, B_6 deficiency could promote tooth decay from within.

If vitamin B_6 deficiency is an important cause of cavities, it's worthwhile to alter our diet. Refined sugar should, of course, be restricted. Aside from containing no B_6, sucrose is a preferred food for cavity-causing bacteria. Why is natural sugarcane, which contains tooth-destroying sucrose, also so rich in vitamin B_6? Perhaps this is nature's way of maintaining the delicate balance between health and disease. Another way we can prevent B_6 deficiency is to avoid vitamin B_6 antagonists. Foods fried in vegetable oil at high temperatures will increase the body's need for B_6. FD&C Yellow No. 5 (tartrazine) should also be avoided, since this food dye is broken down by the body into a hydrazine compound. Potato chips are another culprit. Not only are they made from overheated vegetable oils, but they may contain up to 160 parts per million of maleic hydrazide, a suspected B_6 antagonist.

Tooth decay probably has many different causes. As we continue to search for other causes and more-effective means of prevention, we shouldn't ignore the evidence we already have that vitamin B_6 can be safe and effective in preventing cavities.

Chapter

Chinese Restaurant Syndrome 17

Jeff Miller, a 44-year-old executive, and his wife, Sally, had never eaten much Chinese food, so they thought they would try the Chinese restaurant that had recently opened near their home. After savoring the won ton soup, the egg rolls, the chicken chow mein and the fortune cookies, Mr. and Mrs. Miller paid their compliments to the chef and headed for home.

No sooner had Jeff started the car than he began to feel strange. At first he noticed only a vague tingling sensation in his upper back. The feeling rapidly grew worse, however, and soon he was experiencing severe chest pain. He began to perspire, and he felt his heart pounding rapidly inside his chest. He became extremely thirsty, and he felt as though his head had a tight band wrapped around it. By that time Jeff was really scared. All he could think about was the heart attack his longtime friend from college had suffered only two months before. Was it Jeff's turn now?

Sally quickly drove her husband to the nearest hospital emergency room, where he was immediately placed on a cardiac monitor. After a while his symptoms began to subside, and subsequent tests showed no problem with his heart. What, then, had caused these frightening symptoms? After carefully questioning the Millers, an astute doctor in the emergency room figured out the answer. Jeff was a victim of the Chinese restaurant syndrome—an unusually severe reaction to monosodium glutamate (MSG).

Although such a strong reaction to MSG is uncommon, lesser symptoms occur frequently. A dose of 3 grams of MSG, the amount in a single bowl of won ton soup, was enough to provoke unpleasant symptoms in 22 percent of a test group of healthy people.[1] The most common symptoms were tingling and weakness around the face, temples, upper back, neck and arms, accompanied by a feeling of warmth. In some cases heart palpitations and a sensation of pressure in the chest developed. Other symptoms caused by MSG include a sensation of tightness over the scalp, numb legs, heavy eyelids, pain behind the eyes, headaches, anxiety, flushed skin, mood changes and an urgent need to urinate. Some individuals develop intense thirst, abdominal discomfort, as well as nausea and vomiting after eating foods that contain MSG.[1-4] These symptoms can be frightening, especially if you don't know why they're happening.

MSG has produced arrhythmias—potentially dangerous heart rhythm disturbances. In one patient this arrhythmia lasted for hours and triggered a long period in which the heart was unable to pump an adequate amount of blood.[5] MSG has also caused children to have attacks that resemble epileptic seizures.[6]

What is this chemical that causes so many health problems? MSG is chemically related to glutamic acid, an amino acid normally present in many foods and in the body. Glutamic acid, glutamate and MSG may, for all practical purposes, be considered interchangeable, since the body can easily convert each of these molecules into the other, depending on its needs.

Glutamate participates in a number of the body's essential functions. It forms one of the building blocks of protein molecules and is also present in large amounts in the brain. This chemical appears to play two separate roles in regulating the brain's activity. Glutamate itself tends to stimulate certain portions of the nervous system. And one of glutamate's by-products—gamma-aminobutyric acid (GABA)—acts as a nervous-system inhibitor. Together with its by-products, glutamic acid seems to be important for "fine-tuning" the brain's activity. It is also an energy source for brain tissue.[7]

Glutamic acid also appears to have some therapeutic value. It has reportedly improved the intelligence of some mentally retarded children[8] and reduced the frequency of seizures in some epileptic patients.[9] Glutamic acid in the form of glutamic acid hydrochloride stimulates the stomach to produce its normal digestive juices, too.[10] When used as a supplement at mealtime, it improves digestion in people whose stomachs do not produce enough hydrochloric acid.

MSG's flavor-enhancing effect may be related to its general ability to stimulate the nervous system. Perhaps it stimulates nerve cells that affect the sense of taste. Regardless of how it works, MSG does improve the taste of food and is therefore used extensively by the food industry and by restaurants.

Because MSG occurs naturally in food and in the body, its safety has usually been taken for granted. In fact, the Food and Drug Administration includes MSG on the GRAS (Generally Recognized as Safe) list for food additives, yet there is little doubt that MSG can trigger disturbing symptoms in some people.

MSG's Shock Effects

How could a naturally occurring nutrient produce so many uncomfortable symptoms? How could a molecule that performs crucial biochemical functions cause adverse reactions in such a large percentage of the population? There is actually an important difference between the MSG present in natural food and that used as an additive. The former can be absorbed into the bloodstream only as fast as the digestive process breaks it down from food protein, so the glutamic acid in food enters the system in a "time-release" fashion. Commercial MSG, on the other hand, is already broken down before it's put into the food. As such, it's capable of "shocking" the system with a large number of MSG molecules all at once.

It's not unusual for a single compound to produce different effects, depending on whether it enters the blood slowly or with explosive rapidity. Glucose, for example, is a refined sugar that can be derived from cornstarch. When ingested in its pure form by a sugar-sensitive person, glucose may cause fatigue, weakness, anxiety and sweating. When the same amount of glucose is taken in by eating an ear of corn, the slow release of sugar prevents such symptoms from occurring. In the same way, pure refined MSG may cause symptoms, while naturally occurring glutamic acid does not.

Unfortunately, although MSG reactions are quite common, they often go unrecognized. There are two reasons for this: First, many of us aren't aware that MSG can cause such a wide variety of symptoms. An MSG reactor may present the doctor with a long list of seemingly unrelated complaints. Patients with multiple symptoms that don't "fit together" according to standard medical textbooks are often considered hypochondriacs and are told the problem is all in their head. Thus, the very nature of MSG intolerance makes it likely to be passed off as a psychosomatic illness.

Second, most of us associate MSG only with Chinese restaurants and fail to realize that it's added to countless other foods. If someone gets sick before the waiter has had a chance to clear the won ton soup bowl from the table, then the cause is obvious, but MSG may also be hidden in just about any food. At last count, more than 200,000 tons of MSG were being produced every year.[1] It's often present in seasoned salts, soy sauce, bouillons, gravy mixes, meat bases, cheese chips, crackers, TV dinners, dried and canned soups, hors d'oeuvres and numerous precooked and frozen packaged foods. Some restaurant owners admit that MSG is used to enhance the flavor of nearly every dish they serve. To heighten the confusion, manufacturers are not required by law to list MSG on the labels of foods such as salad dressings and mayonnaise.[1]

How can you determine whether your symptoms are due to MSG? There are several clues. If symptoms occur less than 15 minutes or more than an hour after the beginning of the meal, it's unlikely that MSG is involved. MSG reactions usually begin 15 minutes to half an hour from the start of the meal and last about 45 minutes.[11] Occasionally an MSG headache will persist for a day or two. If any other of your symptoms lasts an entire day, it is probably not due to MSG. If a suspected food causes problems at the beginning, but not at the end of the meal, then MSG may be the culprit. For some reason, this chemical rarely causes symptoms unless it is eaten on an empty stomach.[1] Perhaps mixing MSG with food slows down the rate of absorption to the point where the additive can no longer "shock" the system. If symptoms occur in restaurants but not when the same food is prepared fresh at home, then suspect MSG.

If you believe MSG is making you ill, try eliminating for a brief period all foods that might possibly contain it. If your symptoms disappear, there is a good chance you are sensitive to this chemical. Even after this test, you may not be able to tell whether you're reacting to the MSG or to some other ingredient. Since overprocessed food may be rather tasteless, it is often sweetened with large amounts of sugar and "enhanced" with MSG. Overprocessed foods may also turn a different color than the same natural food. Manufacturers therefore add artificial coloring to make the final product appear natural. When you eliminate all the MSG from your diet, you may also be cutting out a substantial amount of sugar and additives at the same time. If you are one of the many people who react adversely to these additives, then cutting out all MSG may relieve your symptoms. Improvement on such a diet does not prove you are sensitive to MSG, however.

If you are not sure what you have been reacting to, an MSG challenge test might be worthwhile. This should be done only under the supervision of your doctor, since MSG will on rare occasions produce a serious reaction. Ask a friend to prepare two glasses of tomato juice and add a teaspoon of MSG to one of them. (In order to minimize psychological factors, it's best that you don't know which glass contained the MSG until after the test is completed.) Drink each glass on an empty stomach at a different time. Nearly all MSG-sensitive people react to this dose.[2] If the MSG drink produces typical symptoms and the plain tomato juice doesn't, the problem has been solved.

After you have determined that MSG is causing your difficulty, the only foolproof treatment is to stay away from it. Unfortunately, this may be easier said than done. In my experience, patients who have found it necessary to avoid MSG completely often feel isolated. They are afraid to eat at restaurants or at a friend's home, and they may even feel deprived, since they can't buy so many common supermarket items. For some, "MSG neurosis" is as big a problem as the reaction itself.

Preventing an MSG Reaction

It is, of course, advisable for MSG reactors to avoid this chemical whenever reasonably possible. Fortunately, there's a simple way for some people to reduce or even eliminate MSG sensitivity without avoiding the compound completely. There is now good evidence that vitamin B_6 supplements will cure MSG intolerance in many cases.

Several years ago, Karl Folkers, Ph.D., a pioneer in vitamin B_6 research, postulated that the reason some people react to MSG is that they are deficient in vitamin B_6. Earlier animal studies[12] tended to support Dr. Folkers's theory. These studies showed that B_6 deficiency impairs the body's ability to break down MSG. In one experiment, young rats were given large amounts of this food additive. Rats that were also fed a B_6-deficient diet ended up with higher levels of glutamate in their blood than those given adequate amounts of B_6. The elevated levels of glutamate in the deficient rats appeared to be due to the vitamin B_6 deficiency.[13] There are two enzymes that break down MSG: glutamic oxalacetic transaminase (GOT) and glutamic pyruvic transaminase (GPT). Neither of them can function normally without adequate amounts of B_6. In the B_6-deficient rats, GOT and GPT activity were below normal. These animals had accumulated MSG because the enzymes that break it down could not function efficiently.

If the same process occurs in humans, MSG intolerance might be associated with or even caused by B_6 deficiency. To test this hypothesis, Folkers and co-workers measured B_6 levels in 158 students.[14] The 27 students with the lowest levels were studied further. Each of these students was challenged at separate times with MSG and a placebo. Neither the students nor those administering the test solutions knew which solution contained the MSG. Twelve students reacted to MSG and 15 did not.

The next step in Dr. Folkers's experiment was to determine whether B_6 supplements would affect symptoms. The 12 students who had reacted to MSG were assigned randomly to one of two treatment groups: pyridoxine (50 milligrams daily) or a placebo. Again, no one knew during the test period whether or not he was being given B_6. As it turned out, 9 students had received B_6 and 3 had been given a placebo. After the 12-week period, each student was rechallenged with MSG. Of the 9 in the B_6 group, 8 no longer reacted, whereas all 3 of the students given a placebo continued to have symptoms. The effect of B_6 was considered statistically significant—in other words, the probability that these results might have occurred by chance was less than 1 in 100.[14] Dr. Folkers's study demonstrated clearly that vitamin B_6 will in many cases eliminate symptoms due to MSG ingestion.

Several questions still need to be answered concerning the relationship between vitamin B_6 and MSG intolerance, however. Why did one subject taking B_6 supplements continue to react? Did her body simply need unusually large doses of B_6 in order to function normally, or were there other factors involved? Of the 27 students with the lowest levels of vitamin B_6, why did only 12 react to MSG, while the other 15 tolerated it with no problem? Perhaps the level of B_6 in the blood does not always reflect accurately what is going on in the other tissues. Is it possible that the MSG reactors had lower levels of B_6 in the nervous system than the nonreactors had? Only further research will tell.

Another question that is not yet resolved is whether Dr. Folkers's research applies to everyone or only to people with low levels of vitamin B_6. The only people challenged with MSG in Dr. Folkers's study were those determined in advance to be low in B_6. This group included less than 20 percent of the original group of students. Would any of the students with higher B_6 levels have reacted to MSG? If so, would B_6 supplements have helped? B_6 will not necessarily help everyone.

When B₆ Can't Help

I consulted with M.P., a 36-year-old woman who suffered from severe symptoms whenever she ate foods containing MSG. On one occasion, within 15 minutes of eating hors d'oeuvres and an egg roll at a Chinese restaurant, her heart began to pound extremely rapidly and she had an uncomfortable tingling sensation in her fingers. She also felt as if the blood were rushing out of her head. Another time she experienced such severe palpitations and light-headedness that she was rushed to the nearest emergency room. M.P. developed these reactions whenever she ate at a certain restaurant. However, the same foods prepared at home did not produce a reaction. When she asked the restaurant owner about MSG, he admitted that this chemical was added to every dish he served. M.P. could prevent a reaction to these foods if she ate something before going to the restaurant. This fact and the pattern of her symptoms strongly suggested MSG intolerance. We never proved the diagnosis, because M.P. would not agree to an MSG challenge test. She had already learned to avoid this additive, and she did not feel it was worth triggering another severe attack just to prove a point. Nevertheless, we were both convinced she had been reacting to MSG.

Every day for two years, M.P. had been taking a high-potency B-complex vitamin that contained 100 milligrams of B_6. It's unlikely that this patient was deficient in B_6, because she was taking 50 times the Recommended Dietary Allowance (RDA) for this vitamin. Still, she was apparently reacting severely to MSG.

Thus, it appears that B_6 supplements will not prevent MSG reactions in all cases. We never found out whether larger doses would have helped M.P., because she developed insomnia and a "spacey" feeling every time she increased her dose of B_6.

It is not clear why B_6 helps some individuals while others continue to react to MSG. The biochemical events that lead to MSG intolerance are probably very complex. There may be other abnormalities involved in addition to vitamin B_6 deficiency. For example, some allergic reactions mimic MSG-induced symptoms. Most of the MSG we consume is made from corn or sugar beets, which are very allergenic foods. Even though

MSG is a relatively pure product, it may still contain some impurities derived from the corn or beets. MSG can provoke quite severe symptoms in people allergic to these impurities.

Someone who has not seen it happen may find it hard to believe that such a small amount of a food can cause trouble, but these reactions are not uncommon. It seems that the speed with which an allergenic substance is absorbed is at least as important as, and possibly more important than, the amount absorbed. A food-sensitive person tends to react more severely to rapidly absorbed sources of that food, like alcoholic beverages. Corn syrup and beet sugar are often the worst offenders for people allergic to corn or beets.[15] Since MSG is also absorbed relatively quickly, it's likely to trigger symptoms in corn- or beet-allergic people.

It's clear that B_6 supplements can't help all MSG-sensitive people. Nevertheless, Dr. Folkers has shown that some people do lose their sensitivity when they take 50 milligrams of B_6 daily. Fortunately, that dose doesn't appear to be dangerous. A therapeutic trial with B_6 may therefore be worthwhile for anyone who develops symptoms after MSG exposure. Of course, you should consult with a nutrition-oriented doctor before embarking on any high-dose vitamin program.

What's MSG Doing in Our Food?

In addition to scientific questions, the use of MSG raises certain philosophical and social issues. Many of us remember reports in the late 1960's that MSG injections produced brain damage in young animals. At that time, this chemical was being added to many baby foods. Consumer advocates argued that the safety of MSG for babies had not been proved. Furthermore, they charged, MSG was being added solely for the benefit of the parents, since babies don't need flavor enhancers in their food. The publicity surrounding these issues eventually led to the removal of MSG from baby food.

Now that our infants have been spared the possible risks of an unnecessary food additive, the time has come for us to examine the use of MSG in general. We must ask ourselves and our food manufacturers why half a billion pounds of MSG must be dumped into the world food supply every year. Is our processed food of such poor quality that it is unpalatable without a flavor enhancer? Have our taste buds been so dulled by a steady diet of sugar and salt that we cannot taste "unenhanced" flavors?

Aside from the obvious symptoms it produces in susceptible persons, and aside from the fact that many foods containing this additive are nutritionally undesirable for other reasons, is MSG really harmful? So far, no one has proved that there are any long-term dangers of MSG. That's not to say that dangers don't exist. Ingestion of small amounts of MSG over a long period could conceivably produce subtle changes in our bodies. So it's a good idea to avoid this additive unless it's needed to treat mental retardation, alcoholism or other medical problems. Could we prevent the potential dangers of MSG by increasing the amount of B_6 in our diets? At present the answer to this question is unknown. It seems logical, however, that when we consume excessive amounts of MSG, our bodies will need more B_6, since the vitamin is required to metabolize MSG.[12]

We do know that vitamin B_6 will in some cases prevent Chinese restaurant syndrome. Since it's quite difficult in today's fast-food society to stay away from this additive completely, a B_6 supplement may be the solution for many of the estimated 50 million people who cannot tolerate MSG.

Chapter
Asthma 18

For most of us, breathing comes naturally—we take it for granted. For the approximately 9 million Americans with asthma, however, taking a breath of air is often a major effort and, at times, a desperate struggle.

Breathing was designed to be simple and effortless. Normally, inhaled air passes easily from the nose or mouth into the trachea (the windpipe). From there it proceeds to the smaller, progressively branching airways in the lungs called bronchioles. Finally, it enters the millions of tiny bubble-shaped structures known as alveoli, where vital oxygen is extracted and carbon dioxide waste is expelled. Since this cycle must be repeated more than 10,000 times a day, we are lucky indeed that breathing requires little conscious effort.

For the asthmatic, this intricate network of branching airways can malfunction at any time. When an attack occurs (often with little warning), the bronchial passages spasm, clamping down so hard that they restrict airflow. In an acute attack, the frightened asthmatic may find himself red-faced, gasping for air, wheezing loudly and coughing violently in an effort to expel the mucus that blocks his narrowed airways. If he is lucky, the attack soon settles down. Too often, however, the asthmatic's struggle to breathe continues to the point of exhaustion, and he is forced to resort to the hospital emergency room for an adrenaline injection. At other times he may suffer for days or weeks with a less serious, but quite annoying, tightness in the chest, wheezing, coughing and congestion.

Though asthma is not uncommon among adults, children are its prime sufferers. Asthma usually begins in childhood, often before the age of three. Young asthmatics may grow up with constant fear of attacks, feelings of inferiority and severe restrictions in life-style or diet. They're plagued by continued dependence on parents, doctors and drugs. Fortunately, most of these children outgrow their symptoms by the time they become teenagers. Those who do not may be doomed to a lifetime of breathing problems. Even the ones who do escape are often left with permanent emotional scars from their years of illness.

Few people ever die from asthma. Instead, the disease takes its toll in the form of physical and emotional suffering, loss of productivity and enormous medical expenses. While modern drugs do provide some relief for the majority of asthmatics, far too many remain ill despite the best that doctors have to offer. Vitamin B_6 is not a panacea, but it does offer a ray of hope.

Attack Triggers

The common denominator among asthmatics is that their bronchial passages tend to overreact to certain stimuli. No one knows why some people are hypersensitive and not others. We do know what kinds of stimuli tend to trigger bronchial spasms. The list includes pollens, molds, animal dander, insects, house dust, foods, food additives, various fumes and chemicals, and respiratory infections. Asthma appears to be hereditary in some cases, but many times the cause is never found.

The first principle of asthma therapy is to avoid the attack triggers. For some asthmatics, merely keeping the house free of dust may eliminate symptoms. Others must avoid certain foods. When the trigger cannot be avoided completely, as with pollens or multiple sensitivities, desensitization therapy (allergy shots) may bring relief.

The second principle of therapy is to drink a lot of fluids. Asthmatics tend to become dehydrated because large amounts of fluid are lost through the lungs during the rapid, labored breathing of asthma. Also, in their struggle to breathe, asthmatics find it difficult to pause long enough to drink. Dehydration aggravates asthma, drying up bronchial mucus secretions, which then further obstruct the already narrowed airways. Some doctors advise asthmatics to drink 8 ounces of water every waking hour.

Most asthmatics receive some sort of drug therapy to relax the muscles that squeeze the bronchi or reduce their hypersensitivity. Unfortunately, drugs often cause side effects—including nausea, vomiting, headaches, diarrhea, heart palpitations, cardiac rhythm disturbances, insomnia and seizures. Some of the medicines lose their effectiveness with time, and after a certain point they could even make the asthma worse. The cortisonelike drugs reserved for the most severe cases can even leach calcium from the bones, promote fungus infections in the bronchi and suppress the adrenal glands. Finally, many asthmatics continue to suffer even on the most potent drugs. While some useful advances in asthma therapy have been made during the past decade, we still need more-effective and less-toxic approaches to treatment. For some asthmatics, treatment with B6 appears to be an important new breakthrough.

The Role of B6

One of the first suggestions that pyridoxine might be related to asthma came in 1975. Using a tryptophan load test (see chapter 1), Platon J. Collipp, M.D., and his colleagues in the Department of Pediatrics at the Nassau County Medical Center in East Meadow, New York, discovered evidence of vitamin B6 deficiency in five children with bronchial asthma.[1] Interestingly, this vitamin deficiency seemed to be more than simply a dietary lack. In fact, these children had to take 100 milligrams of pyridoxine a day, or 50 times the Recommended Dietary Allowance (RDA), before their tryptophan metabolism even approached normal levels. There was obviously something unusual about the biochemistry of asthmatic children that caused them to need 50 times as much pyridoxine as other children. Conceivably, the disease itself could have led to an increased requirement. Or perhaps these children were born with vitamin B6 dependency—an abnormally large need for pyridoxine that, if unsatisfied, could predispose them to developing asthma. This possibility is not farfetched—there are at least half a dozen other pyridoxine-dependency disorders in which massive doses of B6 are necessary for the body to function normally (see chapter 1).

Could pyridoxine dependency also be a cause of asthma in some children? I believe that it could because one of the body's defenses against asthma is epinephrine (adrenaline), and inadequate levels of B_6 might stop the body from producing enough of this hormone.

To test whether B_6 could help asthma, Dr. Collipp recruited 76 children with moderate or severe asthma. Each child was given either vitamin B_6 (200 milligrams a day) or a placebo for five months. The group receiving the vitamin fared better in a number of ways: They required significantly less cortisone, suffered less wheezing, coughing and chest tightness, and generally breathed more easily than the children taking the placebo. In addition, the B_6-treated group had fewer asthma attacks throughout the study, although this improvement was statistically significant only during two of the five months. In cases where the vitamin worked, positive changes were usually noticeable within one month of beginning treatment.

Psychological factors can, of course, contribute to an improvement or worsening of asthma. Any new drug, even a worthless one, would probably help some asthmatics by exerting a placebo effect. By giving half the children a placebo and using the double-blind method, Collipp *proved* that the benefits of pyridoxine were truly due to the vitamin and not to psychological factors.

How much can asthmatics hope for with B_6? Though it's certainly not a cure-all, the vitamin does appear to be an important addition to the fight against asthma. Any improvements that result from pyridoxine therapy are certainly welcome. Any reduction in cortisone dosage should reduce the long-term dangers of this powerful drug. Vitamin B_6 is relatively nontoxic, so it can be tried without fear of major side effects and is unlikely to interact with other medications.

The relationship between vitamin B_6 and hydrazines may also be relevant here (see chapter 1). Are some asthmatics, because of their biochemical makeup, especially sensitive to the B_6-depleting action of hydrazine compounds? Would avoiding hydrazines help some asthmatics? We know that tartrazine (FD&C Yellow No. 5), a commonly used food coloring, is capable of triggering asthmatic attacks. Tartrazine is converted by the body into 4-sulphophenylhydrazine, a hydrazine molecule. While tartrazine is generally thought to trigger asthma through an allergic reaction, it may also work by interfering with B_6 metabolism. Tartrazine causes chronic urticaria (hives) in some people, and some doctors suspect that FD&C Yellow No. 5 may cause systemic lupus erythematosus, a serious autoimmune disease, as well (see chapter 10).

Hundreds of prescription drugs and countless foods contain this chemical, so even the most conscientious among us have a difficult time avoiding it completely. Will extra B_6 help reduce the toxic effects of this ever-present dye? It's certainly worth trying to find out.

All asthmatic children deserve a vitamin B_6 trial. With their doctor's approval, they might take B_6 supplements for a month or so. If the doctor sees no improvement, stop the therapy and nothing will have been lost. Adult asthmatics could also give B_6 a try, although there are no scientific data on its effectiveness for adults. As with all nutritional therapy, vitamin B_6 should be used *only under the supervision of a competent physician*.

Chapter

Other 19
Ailments

So far, we have discussed how vitamin B$_6$ can prevent or relieve a wide range of major medical problems. Here are a variety of other disorders that have also responded to B$_6$.

Fatigue and Weakness

Vitamin B$_6$ deficiency appears to be one of the many different causes, nutritional and otherwise, of fatigue. In one study, 19 people who complained of chronic exhaustion were given pyridoxine tablets, 20 milligrams twice a day, and a placebo, each for seven days. Some of these patients had already tried a wide variety of other remedies for their fatigue, but nothing worked. Vitamin B$_6$ helped all but one.[1] Most of the patients remarked that they felt considerably better during the week on B$_6$ than when they were taking the placebo. While B$_6$ deficiency is obviously not the only cause of tiredness, it would be wise to include this vitamin in an overall nutrition program for people suffering from chronic fatigue.

Vitamin B$_6$ has also been effective for certain types of muscle weakness, including the weakness that develops because of an overactive thyroid gland,[2] and for a disorder known as pseudohypertrophic muscular dystrophy.[3] Some athletes and body builders use vitamin B$_6$ as

173

part of a nutritional program to build stronger muscles, but there is little scientific evidence that B_6 can increase either the strength or size of muscles in healthy people.

Vertigo

Vertigo is a feeling of dizziness or giddiness, a sensation that the room is spinning around. This common complaint has many different causes, some of which are serious. Anyone suffering from repeated episodes of vertigo should be evaluated by a physician, preferably an ear, nose and throat specialist.

In 1947 two physicians from Chicago began experimenting with pyridoxine to treat vertigo. They gave this vitamin to 47 patients with Ménière's disease, a syndrome that includes vertigo, hearing loss and ringing in the ears. Fifteen of these patients had previously failed to improve with other treatments but responded to pyridoxine. Three others didn't improve with B_6 therapy, and many others gradually improved, but it wasn't clear whether B_6 was responsible. These doctors gave vitamin B_6 to 23 other people who had vertigo due to unknown causes. The vitamin was frequently effective in these cases as well. The doctors found that intravenous injections of pyridoxine relieved symptoms more rapidly than oral treatment.[4]

Drugs such as meclizine (sold under the brand names Antivert or Bonine) often relieve the symptoms but may also cause drowsiness and dryness of the mouth. If vitamin B_6 is effective for vertigo, its lack of side effects would make it the preferred treatment in many cases. A double-blind study is needed to determine whether the benefits attributed to B_6 are real or a placebo effect.

Peptic Ulcers

Many factors contribute to the development of peptic ulcers (of the stomach and duodenum), including stress, eating habits and excessive alcohol consumption. Vitamin B_6 deficiency may also be a factor, at least in gastric (stomach) ulcers. A team of Australian doctors measured vitamin B_6 levels in the blood serum of patients with peptic ulcers.[5] The levels were below normal in 28 of 30 people with a gastric ulcer, but in only 1 of 14 with a duodenal ulcer. These data show a strong association between vitamin B_6 deficiency and gastric ulcers.

As I've already mentioned, vitamin B_6 is the coenzyme for lysyl oxidase, an enzyme that helps strengthen connective tissue. When this enzyme functions well, the stomach wall becomes more resistant to the physical and emotional stresses that promote ulcer formation, which means that vitamin B_6 is a resistance factor against gastric ulcers. Conversely, deficiency of this vitamin could contribute to the development of gastric ulcers.

Scientists performed an experiment with mice to determine whether B_6 does in fact help prevent gastric ulcers. When mice are physically restrained so they can't move at all, they become so stressed that they develop stomach ulcers. In this study, some of the mice were given an injection of pyridoxine (1.11 milligrams per kilogram of body weight) before being immobilized. Only 10 percent of the injected mice developed ulcers, compared with 50 percent of the control group, which was injected with water.[6]

Vitamin B_6 and the Skin

When we think of nutrients to promote healthy skin, vitamins A and E, zinc and essential fatty acids usually come to mind. There is evidence that vitamin B_6 also is useful for certain skin disorders. Perhaps some of the benefits of B_6 therapy are due to its interactions with these other nutrients, but B_6 also appears to play a direct role in maintaining healthy skin.

Acne

A report from 1942 suggests that vitamin B_6 may be useful in treating acne.[7] Shortly after pyridoxine became available in pure form, Norman Jolliffe, M.D., and colleagues tested its effect on university students with persistent, severe acne. These students had been suffering with acne for up to ten years, and many had run the gamut of available treatments with little success. Twenty-eight of 37 students improved while taking B_6, and in 9 cases the skin completely cleared up. Some students found that their oily skin cleared up to the point of actual dryness. The effective dose varied from 50 to 250 milligrams a day.

(Doses higher than 50 milligrams a day should not be used without a doctor's advice.) Acne often improves whenever any new treatment is tried, so it's difficult to tell whether the results reported by Dr. Jolliffe were more than a placebo effect.

Many women find that their acne gets much worse just before their period. In one study of 106 teenage girls whose acne usually worsened premenstrually, 72 were helped by taking 50 milligrams of B_6 daily the week before and during their period.[8] Most of the girls stated that their flare-ups were reduced by about 50 to 75 percent. A more recent study failed to confirm the reported benefits of B_6 in premenstrual acne,[9] but since only 9 girls were treated with this vitamin, it's difficult to draw firm conclusions.

Seborrheic Dermatitis

Vitamin B_6 appears to be useful in some cases of seborrheic dermatitis. Persons with this common skin problem, frequently referred to as "seborrhea" or "dandruff," have oily, reddened, scaly lesions on the face, scalp or other areas of the body. In 1941 Paul György, M.D., the man who discovered vitamin B_6, noted that seborrhealike skin lesions developed in rats that were fed a diet low in B_6.[10] Other doctors observed that seborrheic dermatitis improved greatly in six pregnant women after they took B_6 supplements.[11] In another study, injections of pyridoxine (25 to 100 milligrams) produced striking improvements in some people with seborrheic dermatitis, while others didn't improve at all.[12] Apparently, vitamin B_6 deficiency was one factor, though not the only one, causing these skin lesions.

In 1952 A. William Schreiner, M.D., and associates reported an interesting new discovery.[13] Dr. Schreiner treated 25 patients with seborrheic dermatitis of the "sicca" type (red, dry scales on the scalp hairline, eyebrows, ears, nose and lips) with an ointment containing 10 milligrams of pyridoxine per gram. The lesions cleared in 22 of the 25 patients. In some patients the skin cleared up as quickly as five days from the time the ointment was first applied. When skin lesions were treated with a placebo (the same ointment without the B_6), they didn't improve. There was only "questionable improvement" when vitamin B_6 was given by mouth or by injection. Since the vitamin had to be applied directly to the skin to be effective, those with seborrheic dermatitis probably had a metabolic defect in the skin that increased their local requirement for vitamin B_6. People with moist or oozing forms of seborrhea didn't respond to the B₆ ointment, and some cases even got worse. Apparently, there is more than one cause of seborrheic dermatitis. In infants, these skin lesions sometimes respond to the B-vitamin biotin.[14] I have also seen linseed oil, a source of essential fatty acids, produce striking improvements in some chronic cases of dandruff. Perhaps other nutritional factors are also related to this chronic skin condition.

Vitamin B₆ ointment is available at many natural-food stores at a concentration of 50 milligrams per gram. While this ointment doesn't work every time, it's often effective, especially for dry, scaly lesions of the scalp.

Light Sensitivity

Some people are extremely sensitive to sunlight, developing itching or rashes after even short exposures to the sun. Sometimes this photosensitivity is a sign of another illness, such as lupus erythematosus (see chapter 10). In other instances, light sensitivity is a side effect of a prescription drug. In many cases, the cause is never discovered.

In 1963 Edward H. Mandel, M.D., a New York City physician, reported a novel treatment for photosensitivity: vitamin B₆.[15] Dr. Mandel was aware that many people with light-induced skin eruptions have abnormal tryptophan metabolism, an indication that they might be deficient in B₆. He prescribed vitamin B₆ for seven patients who suffered from itching or skin eruptions whenever they went out in the sun. In two of these people, a dose of 150 to 200 milligrams taken 30 minutes before sun exposure completely prevented the reaction from occurring. In others, the vitamin was effective, but only at a dosage of 100 milligrams every hour for nine hours. Interestingly, in one patient, this once-an-hour B₆ treatment taken for only one day protected her against the sun for a full two weeks. Dr. Mandel found that the total dosage of B₆ wasn't as important as how it was taken. For example, some patients who were protected by 100 milligrams an hour for nine hours found that 200 milligrams of B₆ a day for a week didn't protect them at all. Once again, I want to caution you that these large amounts of B₆ should not be taken without the guidance of a physician.

Herpes Gestationis

Herpes gestationis is a rare skin disorder that some women develop during pregnancy. The term *herpes* denotes blisters occurring in a cluster, and *gestationis* refers to pregnancy. The blisters that develop in herpes gestationis can cause severe itching. Aside from being uncomfortable and unsightly, there is evidence that these skin lesions contribute to an increase in fetal mortality. Most dermatologists prescribe cortisonelike drugs (such as prednisone) for herpes gestationis, but these drugs pose some risk for both the mother and the fetus. Several doctors have found that vitamin B_6 is a safe and extremely effective alternative to treat this problem.[16,17] The dosages needed to produce good results varied from 50 to 4,000 milligrams a day (anyone considering taking more than 50 milligrams a day should consult a doctor first). One doctor observed that B_6 worked better when injected than when taken by mouth. Craig G. Burkhart, M.D., of Toledo, Ohio, has remarked on the "amazing success" with which he had used B_6 in one case.

Epilepsy

About three decades ago, an infant formula inadvertently deficient in vitamin B_6 was being sold in the United States. Many children who consumed this formula developed epileptic seizures that disappeared when they took B_6 supplements or changed to another formula.[18] Animal studies had already demonstrated that B_6-deficient diets could cause convulsions. This new observation demonstrated that some cases of human epilepsy also may be related to this vitamin.

Vitamin B_6 deficiency severe enough to cause seizures is uncommon among those who consume a reasonably well-balanced diet. However, some people have what's known as pyridoxine-dependent seizures; that is, they've inherited an unusually large requirement for vitamin B_6 that, if not met, will lead to recurrent seizures. About 50 cases of B_6-dependent epilepsy have been reported in the medical literature. Scientists believe that the genetic defect that causes this problem is in the binding of B_6 to glutamate decarboxylase, an enzyme that converts the amino acid glutamic acid into the neurotransmitter gamma-aminobutyric acid (GABA). The reduced concentration of GABA in the brain that occurs with this genetic abnormality makes the brain more susceptible to seizures. When large amounts of vitamin B_6 are supplied, however, the defective binding is overcome and the seizures are prevented.

Pediatricians have been taught to think of B_6 dependency if the seizures begin within hours after birth and can be controlled only by repeated large doses of vitamin B_6. However, because B_6-dependent epilepsy is so uncommon, doctors tend to forget about it unless the symptoms conform closely to the textbook description. A group of Australian physicians has recently pointed out that pyridoxine dependency must be considered even in children who do not have a typical case.[19] These doctors diagnosed four cases of B₆-dependent epilepsy that were unusual in one or more of the following respects: (1) the symptoms didn't develop immediately after birth; (2) anticonvulsant drugs controlled the seizures for a while; (3) it took a long time for symptoms to recur after B₆ was stopped; and (4) the seizures were not typical of B₆ dependency. So although none of these children fit the classic description, in each case, large doses of vitamin B₆ kept the seizures under control. The Australian doctors suggested that B₆-dependent epilepsy isn't as rare as doctors had previously thought, and that it should be considered in diagnosing any infant with difficult-to-treat epilepsy.

Although vitamin B₆ supplements may help some children with epilepsy, parents should not give their children large amounts of this vitamin without close supervision by a physician. Vitamin B₆ in doses ranging from 80 to 400 milligrams a day has been shown to interfere with some of the commonly used anticonvulsant medications and could therefore make seizures worse if not carefully monitored.[20]

Parkinson's Disease

Parkinson's disease is a neurological disorder that occurs in the middle-aged or the elderly. Its symptoms include hand tremors, rigidity of the face and other portions of the body, and a general slowing of movement. The disease gradually worsens and may eventually become incapacitating.

The symptoms of Parkinson's disease are related in part to a shortage of the neurotransmitter dopamine in certain areas of the brain. Treatment of this disorder has therefore been aimed at increasing dopamine levels in the brain. Dopamine itself is, for some reason, unable to travel into the brain. Doctors use another compound called L-dopa, which can cross the blood-brain barrier and be converted into dopamine once inside the brain. L-dopa usually improves the symptoms of Parkinson's disease, although it isn't a cure.

Although both L-dopa and dopamine are naturally present in the brain and other areas of the body, the conversion of the L-dopa to dopamine requires a B_6-dependent enzyme. Conceivably, B_6 supplements would help patients with Parkinson's disease by increasing this conversion. About 40 years ago, a number of doctors tested this possibility. In one report,[21] six patients were regularly given injections of 50 or 100 milligrams of B_6 over a 19-day to five-month period. Five of these patients showed improvements in posture, gait, coordination and general well-being. In another study, four of nine people improved after receiving B_6 injections, and a few patients treated with B_6 and brewer's yeast also seemed to do better.[22] Other doctors, however, found that vitamin B_6 treatment didn't improve the symptoms of Parkinson's disease.[23,24]

With the discovery that L-dopa was beneficial, interest in using B_6 supplements waned. Indeed, it soon became clear that vitamin B_6 could actually interfere with the therapeutic effect of L-dopa. The vitamin apparently stimulated enzymes outside the brain to convert L-dopa into dopamine, and since dopamine can't get into the brain from the blood, much of the L-dopa was wasted. In one study, B_6 was given to four patients with Parkinson's disease who were taking L-dopa. In three cases, symptoms worsened. The fourth person, who was suffering from side effects of L-dopa overdose, improved.[25] It seemed that B_6 should be limited to the treatment of L-dopa intoxication.

The picture changed somewhat with the discovery of a new drug called carbidopa. This drug (which is, interestingly enough, a hydrazine molecule) influences the metabolism of L-dopa outside, but not inside, the brain. Carbidopa prevents L-dopa from being converted to dopamine. Doctors often prescribe the combination of L-dopa and carbidopa (Sinemet), because carbidopa allows a greater percentage of L-dopa to get into the brain, where it can then be transformed to dopamine.

The discovery of carbidopa has once again raised the possibility that B_6 might help patients with Parkinson's disease. Vitamin B_6 supplements might improve the conversion of L-dopa to dopamine within the brain, while carbidopa prevents B_6 from destroying L-dopa on the outside. In other words, extra B_6 taken along with Sinemet could presumably increase the production of dopamine in the brain without reducing the amount of L-dopa available to the brain.[26]

So far there has been little clinical research comparing Sinemet alone to Sinemet plus B_6. We do know, however, that the hydrazine compound carbidopa can promote vitamin B_6 deficiency. In studies at the Massachusetts Institute of Technology, injections of carbidopa into rats depleted vitamin B_6 from various tissues.[27] There is also some indication that L-dopa itself may cause B_6 deficiency.[28] Since B_6 is needed to convert L-dopa to dopamine, deficiency of this vitamin could make Parkinson's disease worse. The most effective treatment for Parkinson's disease may turn out to be a combination of Sinemet and vitamin B_6. Additional research is needed to determine what doses of each compound will give the best results with the fewest unwanted side effects.

Allergy

Nutrition-oriented doctors have been impressed that certain vitamin supplements often take the edge off allergy symptoms. Nutrients such as pantothenate, vitamin C and vitamin B_6 are frequently used for such symptoms as hay fever and chronic nasal congestion. Although not everyone who takes these vitamins finds relief, many people feel that this combination of nutrients works as well as antihistamines. Furthermore, nutritional therapy doesn't cause the annoying side effects, such as dry mucous membranes and drowsiness, that occur with antihistamines.

Vitamin therapy is not widely used for allergies, possibly because there have been few controlled studies documenting its value. Nevertheless, there is some research suggesting that the enthusiastic observations made by a few physicians are valid. In the case of vitamin B_6, studies both in animals and in the test tube point to an "antiallergy" role for this vitamin.

There is a chemical inside the body called histamine, which triggers allergic reactions. This molecule is stored inside specialized white blood cells known as mast cells. When exposed to an allergy-provoking agent such as dust or an offending food, these mast cells explode and release histamine into the system. The so-called "antihistamines" relieve allergies by interfering with the action of histamine. Vitamin B_6 also appears to be an antihistamine of sorts; it changes the structure of histamine by forming a chemical bond with it. Presumably, this altered histamine molecule is no longer capable of provoking an allergic reaction. A group of Polish doctors has suggested that this interaction may be one way of removing excess histamine from the body.[29]

In addition to interfering with histamine, vitamin B_6 appears to block allergies in another way. A group of Cuban doctors found that when they mixed B_6 with mast cells in a test tube, they reduced the cells' tendency to explode.[30] Vitamin B_6 should help prevent allergic reactions from developing by stabilizing the mast cells. Perhaps further research will determine whether this test-tube effect of B_6 applies to real life as well.

A number of years ago, researchers found that vitamin B_6 has a potent effect in blocking allergic reactions in animals. When "sensitized" guinea pigs are given an injection of blood serum taken from a horse, they develop a severe and sometimes fatal allergic reaction known as anaphylactic shock. In one study, guinea pigs were given an injection of pyridoxine (up to 184 milligrams per kilogram of body weight) before receiving the fatal dose of horse serum. The B_6 injection prevented death and reduced the severity of the allergic reaction.[31] The smallest dose of B_6 (28 milligrams per kilogram) failed to prevent anaphylactic shock. This study demonstrated that B_6 in large doses has a powerful effect on the allergy mechanism.

The modern medical approach to allergies consists mainly of antihistamines and cortisonelike drugs. Although these drugs are effective, they can produce bothersome and sometimes serious side effects. Nutrients, on the other hand, when used intelligently, are quite safe and sometimes work just as well as the drugs. In the interest of better medical care, it's imperative that scientists look more closely into the treatment of allergies with nutrients. The optimal dosages and combinations of B_6, pantothenate and vitamin C for the treatment of allergies remain to be determined.

Vitamin B_6 and the Eyes

Vitamin B_6 may have value in an eye disorder known as the sicca syndrome. The term *sicca* means dry, and the syndrome includes dry eyes, resulting from inadequate production of tears. This disorder often plagues the middle-aged and can cause blurring of vision, burning, itching and a sensation of sand in the eyes. People suffering from the sicca syndrome must put artificial tears in their eyes several times a day to minimize these symptoms. At present, orthodox medicine has no effective treatment for this fairly common problem.

Studies in animals have shown that vitamin B_6 deficiency causes decreased tear flow.[32] David F. Horrobin, M.D., Ph.D., has suggested that loss of tear secretion may be related to inadequate formation of a hormonelike compound called prostaglandin E1 (PGE1). This molecule is manufactured by the body from the essential fatty acid linoleic acid by a series of enzymes that are believed to require vitamins B_6 and C.[33]

In order to promote PGE1 production, Dr. Horrobin's associates treated four patients suffering from dry eyes with vitamin B_6 (25 to 50 milligrams a day), vitamin C (2 to 3 grams a day) and evening primrose oil, a rich source of essential fatty acids (two capsules three times a day). All four of these patients noticed an improvement in their eye condition.[34] Because of their good results, Dr. Horrobin's group continued to prescribe this treatment for others with the sicca syndrome. (You should never take such large amounts of these substances without a doctor's supervision.) As of 1981, they had treated 17 people, of whom 10 had shown either substantial improvement or complete resolution of their eye problems.[33]

The work with vitamins B_6, C and evening primrose oil was then extended to patients suffering from Sjögren's syndrome, another disorder of tear secretion associated with arthritis and other symptoms. Sjögren's syndrome is an autoimmune disease in which the body's immune system attacks its own tissues, including the tear-producing glands. A Canadian physician tried Dr. Horrobin's successful remedy in ten patients with Sjögren's syndrome. Unfortunately, none of these patients improved significantly after ten weeks of therapy.[35]

These studies indicate that some people's eyes will improve after treatment with pyridoxine, vitamin C and evening primrose oil, but when the sicca syndrome is associated with Sjögren's syndrome, this remedy doesn't usually work. I'd like to point out that Dr. Horrobin's treatment doesn't always fail with Sjögren's syndrome; one of his colleagues successfully treated a patient with this disorder.

Radiation Sickness

People exposed to large doses of X rays, either accidentally or during cancer therapy, may develop symptoms of radiation sickness, including loss of appetite, nausea and vomiting, and malaise. A number of reports from about four decades ago suggested that vitamin B_6 supplements are an effective means of treating or preventing radiation sickness.[36-38] The usual dose prescribed was in the range of 40 to 100 milligrams a day by mouth. In cases where oral B_6 did not help, intravenous injections usually produced a rapid response.

Today only a few doctors prescribe vitamin B_6 along with radiation therapy. Most physicians who are aware of this treatment believe it's just a placebo. No good controlled studies have been done to substantiate the alleged benefits of B_6. Animal studies, however, have shown that a deficiency of B_6 and other vitamins increases susceptibility to radiation sickness.[39]

Modern man is being exposed to increasing amounts of radiation. Significant sources include diagnostic X rays, contamination from nuclear power plants, X rays from television sets and fallout from atomic weapons testing. Further research should be done to determine whether vitamin B_6 can minimize some of the damaging effects of low-level radiation exposure. If so, we have yet another reason to increase our intake of this important vitamin.

Tetanus

Tetanus is a major cause of infant mortality, particularly in developing countries. Conventional treatment, which includes tetanus antitoxin and antibiotics, has not substantially reduced the death rate from this serious infection. Children afflicted with tetanus develop severe spasms and stiffness in the muscles of the jaw, neck and other parts of the body. These spasms, which are caused by a toxin produced by the tetanus bacterium, can also paralyze the breathing apparatus, leading to pneumonia or death from asphyxiation.

There is some evidence that the tetanus toxin causes muscle spasms by interfering with the neurotransmitter gamma-aminobutyric acid (GABA). As you may recall, a neurotransmitter is a chemical messenger that transmits signals through the nervous system. Since GABA appears to inhibit muscle contractions, any chemical that interferes with this neurotransmitter might promote spasms. GABA is produced from the amino acid glutamic acid by a reaction that requires vitamin B_6. Conceivably, if more B_6 were supplied to a child suffering from tetanus, more GABA would be produced, and muscle spasms might be relieved.

Because of this intriguing possibility that vitamin B_6 might be helpful, a doctor in Tunisia decided to give this vitamin to infants who had developed tetanus.[40] Each child received a daily intramuscular injection of 100 milligrams of pyridoxine until the muscle spasms disappeared. Conventional treatment was also provided. Only 3 of the 20 children died, a mortality rate of 15 percent. The children treated with B_6 also appeared to recover from muscle spasms faster than with conventional treatment alone. One child died several months later, apparently of causes unrelated to tetanus.

These results signal a major advance in the treatment of tetanus in developing countries. Before pyridoxine was used, nearly every Tunisian infant with tetanus died. In other countries around the world where modern medical facilities are not available, the death rate of infants with tetanus ranges from 60 percent to more than 90 percent.

In countries like the United States, which have sophisticated intensive care units and mechanical respirators, the mortality rate is lower but still unacceptably high. Because tetanus is a life-threatening illness and pyridoxine is relatively nontoxic, all chidren with tetanus should be treated with pyridoxine along with conventional therapy.

Part VI

Understanding How B$_6$ Works

Chapter
How to Use 20
B₆ Safely

The evidence I have presented in this book indicates that most Americans should increase their intake of vitamin B_6. B_6 is valuable in preventing and treating a wide range of disorders, and the Recommended Dietary Allowance (RDA) of 2 milligrams a day is simply not enough to promote optimal health for many people. Environmental pollution and modern food processing techniques seem to have greatly increased our need for this important nutrient.

Vitamin B_6 supplements alone are not the answer to disease prevention—they should be part of a comprehensive nutrition program. To start, try reducing your consumption of refined sugar and refined flour, salt, overprocessed foods, additives and fats. Nutritional supplements usually work better when they are backed up by a healthful diet consisting of whole, unprocessed foods. Whenever possible, avoid hydrazines and other antimetabolites found in the food supply and in the environment.

Since nutrients work together as a team, other supplements should generally be taken along with B_6. Most nutritionists believe that large doses of a single B vitamin will cause deficiencies of other members of the B complex. Although there is little scientific research to support this idea, balancing the B vitamins appears to be a sensible thing to do. There may be some exceptions to this rule, however. For example, a few hyperactive children who improved with vitamin B_6 got worse when they took thiamine (vitamin B_1) supplements.[1] Other children who improved with thiamine deteriorated while taking B_6. There may be other interactions between the various B vitamins that have not yet been discovered. It's possible that backing up vitamin B_6 with the entire B complex will in some cases reduce B_6's effectiveness. This possibility has not yet been carefully studied. On the positive side, research indicates that B_6 may work better in the company of magnesium, zinc, vitamin E and essential fatty acids. In some instances, moderate amounts of a combination of these nutrients work at least as well as large doses of any one of them. Before embarking on a nutrition program, you should consult a doctor knowledgeable in the field.

As a result of all the publicity B_6 has been receiving lately, many people are now taking huge quantities of this vitamin every day, often without medical supervision, so it's important to know how safe B_6 really is. The potential hazards of nutritional therapy must be viewed, of course, in the context of the available alternatives. Compared to the traditional drug-and-surgical approach, nutrients are extremely safe. Medical nutritionists have guided hundreds of thousands of Americans back to good health through a program of diet and supplements. What's so exciting about vitamins and minerals is not that they often work better than drugs (they do), but that they can usually be taken without fear of toxicity. Unlike traditional physicians, nutritionists rarely see serious side effects from their prescriptions. The list of severe and sometimes permanent injuries caused by modern medical care, on the other hand, is painful to recite. The advantages of nutritional therapy over traditional medicine are obvious to those who practice this alternative brand of medicine.

Even though nutrients are safer than drugs, we can't afford to be complacent about nutritional therapy. If used unwisely, nutrients may indeed cause harm.

Exercising Caution

Nutritional therapy could cause several kinds of problems: It could tempt people to overemphasize self-diagnosis instead of seeking competent medical advice; certain nutrients can distort the results of some laboratory tests; and some nutrients can be toxic when used improperly.

Let's look at self-diagnosis first. Some people stay away from doctors because they have little faith in modern medicine. They or someone they know may have been a victim of iatrogenic (doctor-induced) disease. Or perhaps they disagree with the drug-oriented philosophy that most doctors have. With all the popular health books and magazines on the market, self-diagnosis and self-treatment is sometimes a tempting alternative to making an appointment with the doctor. Unfortunately, your own diagnosis will frequently be wrong, no matter how closely your symptoms match a description in an article or book. If you treat yourself without really knowing what the problem is, you could overlook a serious but treatable disease.

Suppose, for example, that you have developed numbness, tingling and pain in the thumb and first two fingers of each hand. According to your reading, these resemble early symptoms of the carpal tunnel syndrome, which you know can be treated with vitamin B_6 supplements. But your symptoms could also be caused by a degenerating disc in your spine. Then, too, carpal tunnel syndrome may be an early symptom of hypothyroidism or rheumatoid arthritis. If you treat yourself with B_6 instead of having your symptoms diagnosed correctly, you may delay important medical treatment, such as neck traction or thyroid hormones. Before starting your own nutrition program, get checked out by your doctor to make sure you have no serious health problems. If you are treating an illness nutritionally, make sure your doctor monitors your progress. If you can, find a physician who is knowledgeable about nutrition.

The second problem I mentioned is that some vitamin supplements can distort the results of standard laboratory tests. For example, there is a simple chemical test to detect small amounts of bleeding from the bowel. This test is an important screening tool for early intestinal cancer, diverticulitis or other gastrointestinal diseases. If you are taking several thousand milligrams of vitamin C every day, however, the test may fail to detect blood in the stool. Folate supplements are another example. They can interfere with a common test for pernicious anemia. If you're scheduled for diagnostic tests and you take vitamin C or folate, be sure to inform your doctor. As far as I know, vitamin B_6 doesn't interfere with any diagnostic tests.

The third possible hazard I mentioned comes from the nutrients themselves. Some nutrients, such as vitamins A and D, niacinamide and selenium, can be quite toxic if taken to excess. Even vitamin B_6, a relatively safe vitamin, can cause problems if it's not taken wisely. A recent report of nerve damage in seven people who were taking massive amounts of B_6 underscores the potential dangers of using megavitamins without careful supervision by a professional trained in nutrition.[2]

On the other hand, if B₆ is taken with good judgment, there is little chance of it causing serious harm. Short-term use of B₆ appears to be quite safe, especially if you consult your doctor before taking any more than 50 milligrams a day. Patients suffering from an acute overdose of the antituberculous drug isoniazid have been treated with up to 25 grams (25,000 milligrams) of vitamin B₆ intravenously without adverse effects.[3] Of course, except for treatment of a drug overdose, there is no reason that anyone should have to take such large amounts of B₆.

What about the long-term risks? A few people with inherited vitamin B₆-dependency syndromes have been taking between 200 and 600 milligrams a day for extended periods,[4] and no reports of toxicity have appeared in the medical literature. Some women with premenstrual syndrome have been taking up to 800 milligrams daily without apparent toxic effects.[5] A few patients with recurrent kidney stones due to a defect in oxalate metabolism have taken 1,000 milligrams of B₆ daily for several years. The vitamin improved their kidney function without producing any noticeable toxicity.[6]

Too Much of a Good Thing

Still, the apparent safety of vitamin B₆ in doses several hundred times the RDA can't be construed as evidence that this vitamin is entirely safe at any dose. Any nutrient can be toxic if taken in large enough amounts, and vitamin B₆ is no exception. On August 25, 1983, Herbert Schaumburg, M.D., and colleagues published a report in the *New England Journal of Medicine* titled "Sensory Neuropathy from Pyridoxine Abuse."[2] These doctors had seen patients in whom severe impairment of sensory nerve function occurred while they were taking between 2,000 and 6,000 milligrams of pyridoxine a day. The symptoms typically began with numbness in the feet and instability while walking. This was followed by numbness around the mouth and hands and clumsiness in handling things. In a few cases, nerve biopsies revealed axonal degeneration in the nerve cells. The doctors performed extensive neurological and laboratory tests on each patient and could find no cause for this syndrome besides the supplements. After discontinuing the B₆, all patients gradually improved, although some of them still had slight neurological abnormalities even after two or three years.

Dr. Schaumburg's report was the first to document serious toxicity from vitamin B₆. Of course, the doses that caused nerve damage were far greater than those usually needed to prevent or treat illness. Most of the disorders I have described in this book can be treated with 50 milligrams of B₆ a day, although some people require larger amounts. Nerve damage occurred only at doses of 2,000 milligrams a day or more. Except in very unusual cases, and under a doctor's close supervision, no one should be taking that much vitamin B₆.

Being able to buy megavitamins without a prescription is a mixed blessing. On one hand, the informed consumer can bypass the nutritional ignorance of the medical establishment. On the other hand, easy access to vitamins and minerals increases the likelihood that the misinformed consumer will harm himself. With the increasing publicity surrounding nutritional therapy, more and more people are taking supplements. Some assume that vitamins are completely safe, so if a little bit is good, more might be better. Dr. Schaumburg's report underscores the importance of good judgment and sound medical advice as a part of any nutritional program.

Some doctors have questioned the validity of Dr. Schaumburg's study, since there was no real proof that vitamin B₆ had caused the neurological deficits. The report was based on anecdotal information, the same type of data that traditional doctors reject when used in *support* of vitamin therapy. There are two reasons why Dr. Schaumburg's work must be taken seriously, however. First, no other cause of the nerve damage was found. Second, a similar type of neurological disorder has been produced in animals by feeding them large amounts of pyridoxine.[7] Six of the seven patients who developed problems from B₆ weren't taking any other supplements. Perhaps the high doses of B₆ had produced a deficiency of other B vitamins, which in turn caused the nerve damage. However, in studies where animals were given large amounts of vitamin B₆, no deficiency of any of the other B-complex vitamins occurred.[8] The abnormalities Dr. Schaumburg observed probably were directly attributable to vitamin B₆.

Several other less serious side effects of vitamin B₆ have been reported by some people who take moderate amounts (say, 50 to 200 milligrams a day). They complain of nervousness, insomnia or a feeling of being "wired." Children taking this vitamin may begin wetting their bed or become irritable and more sensitive to sound. According to Bernard Rimland, Ph.D.,[9] these are the symptoms of mild magnesium deficiency. Since B₆ and magnesium work as a team, a B₆ supplement may increase the need for magnesium. These side effects of B₆ therapy can usually be prevented or eliminated by taking additional magnesium.

Many patients report that B_6 makes them urinate more. This may actually be beneficial, since B_6 appears to help the body eliminate excess fluid. This effect generally subsides once the body has been rid of the extra fluid. Since B_6 acts as a diuretic for some people, it may deplete the body of minerals, as other diuretics do. So far, little research has been done in this area. Until the question is settled, it's probably a good idea to take a multiple mineral supplement in conjunction with B_6.

One other possible side effect of vitamin B_6 was reported by French scientists several years ago.[10] These scientists administered a standard intelligence test to student volunteers. Each of the students was then given either vitamin B_6 (100 or 500 milligrams a day) or a placebo for ten days, after which the test was repeated. The results of the study showed that the larger dose of B_6 decreased the students' ability to memorize a series of numbers and letters. The low-dose B_6 group also performed worse than the placebo group, but the results were not statistically significant. This study suggested that large doses of B_6 might impair the ability of students to learn.

I've never heard any patient complain of memory loss while on a comprehensive nutritional program (including several hundred milligrams of B_6). Maybe this side effect of B_6 is prevented when magnesium, zinc and other B vitamins are taken at the same time. On the other hand, the French study measured subtle changes that might not be evident in clinical practice. This possible side effect of vitamin B_6 needs to be looked into further. Studies in animals have confirmed that very large doses of B_6 affect brain function. When rats were fed 200 times the usual amount of B_6, they showed a decrease in general activity and curiosity.[11]

As you can see, vitamin B_6 is not totally harmless. Overdoses of any nutritional product can be dangerous. Apparently, 50 milligrams of B_6 can be taken daily without fear of serious consequences. In most cases, even much larger amounts can be used safely, but *it would be unwise to take more than 50 milligrams a day without medical supervision*.

This warning about potential toxicity isn't meant to discourage you from taking B_6 at all. The thesis of this book is that most of us need more of this vitamin and that some of us need considerably more. With a little bit of homework, common sense and medical advice, you should be able to use this and other nutrients to your advantage, without any risk of serious harm.

Chapter
Directions 21
for Future
Research

The evidence I have reviewed in this book suggests that certain changes in the environment and in our food supply have created a new epidemic, so that some people are now dependent on unusually large doses of vitamin B_6 in order to stay healthy.

The fact that a single vitamin can improve health or relieve illness in so many ways should serve as an example of how great the potential of nutritional therapy is. Vitamin B_6 is only one of a dozen or so different vitamins, and there are at least two dozen other nutrients that play a role in maintaining well-being. If vitamin B_6 alone is so useful, then the possible benefits to be obtained by providing the optimum amounts of all nutrients appear virtually limitless. When combined with proper attention to a healthful diet, food allergies, nutrient absorption, heavy-metal burdens (such as lead and cadmium) and other factors medical nutritionists consider important, the results of nutrient therapy are frequently dramatic. My colleagues in the field and I have become accustomed to hearing patients tell us nearly every day that problems they've had for most of their lives have disappeared after a few weeks or months of therapy. How many traditional doctors can make that statement?

The majority of traditional doctors still turn up their noses at the entire concept of nutritional therapy. Terms such as "quack" and "incompetent" are still gleefully tossed around by specialists in reference to those who dare to believe in this alternative. Nutritionists are frequently criticized for being unscientific and for believing in "anecdotal" information. We are told that the only legitimate way to demonstrate the effectiveness of our treatments is to perform double-blind, placebo-controlled studies. This demand is reminiscent of the Wizard of Oz's requirement that Dorothy and friends bring him the broomstick of the Wicked Witch of the West. Like the Wizard, perhaps they assume that the unobtainable goals they set for us will exasperate us and make us go away. They're wrong. Because nutritional therapy is in many cases a better alternative to medicine as it's currently practiced, it can only become more popular with time. It will soon become clear that the demand for double-blind studies is just a smoke screen put up by those who are satisfied with the status quo.

I am not trying to argue that anecdotal information is more reliable than placebo-controlled studies. Whenever possible, treatments *should* be studied under carefully controlled conditions. The problem is that the practice of nutritional therapy cannot reasonably be tested within the restrictions of this research design. Even if unlimited funds were present for nutrition research, double-blind studies would still be inappropriate in many situations.

Take, for example, a typical diabetic being treated nutritionally. This person would most likely be consuming a high-fiber diet low in sugar and supplemented with brewer's yeast, vitamin C, B complex, additional B_6, vitamin E, magnesium, zinc and perhaps half a dozen other supplements. This program would no doubt be tailored to the special needs of the patient. In trying to prove that this treatment works, one would have to devise an "identical" placebo treatment. How does one begin to fake a high-fiber diet and a tablespoon of brewer's yeast?

And how can one hope to demonstrate by statistical methods a treatment that is by its very nature individualized? Consider the nutritional treatment of chronic diarrhea, for which a wide variety of remedies are used, including eliminating offending food allergens; reducing coffee intake; and taking digestive aids, *L. acidophilus* or folate supplements. Each of these treatments unquestionably works in specific cases, but since none works in the majority of cases, none would be found effective in a small clinical trial. Suppose, for example, that folate deficiency is the cause of diarrhea in 5 percent of cases. Suppose also that 20 percent of people suffering from diarrhea are placebo responders; that is, they improve for a while with any treatment. Out of two groups of 100, 20 would respond to the placebo and 25 to folate. These results wouldn't be statistically significant, and the investigators would wrongly conclude that folate doesn't relieve diarrhea.

The fact is, if traditional doctors rejected every treatment that hasn't been proved by the methods they now worship, their therapeutic arsenal would be decimated. Aspirin has never been shown to relieve pain in a double-blind study, yet everyone knows it works. Bed rest is considered standard treatment for certain back injuries. If we were to try to prove that bed rest helps, we would need a group of placebo-treated patients who wouldn't know whether or not they were in bed! If we really wanted to study the newest anticancer drug properly, we would have to come up with an "inert" placebo that caused hair loss, diarrhea and possibly death. In order to prove whether or not that new surgical technique is helpful, we would have to perform a "sham operation" on half the patients and compare the results. Obviously, doctors make therapeutic decisions all the time on the basis of less-than-perfect data. Why have a double standard where nutritional therapy is concerned?

Good Anecdotes and Bad Ones

Some of the most important advances in medical care have been made as a result of careful observation. Had these observations been rejected out of hand as worthless anecdotal information, medicine would never have progressed. Scientific objectivity and skepticism are virtues, but we must also recognize the difference between a good anecdote and a bad one. "My rheumatoid arthritis improved after I began taking zinc" is a bad anecdote. The symptoms of rheumatoid arthritis are unpredictable, and spontaneous improvements are not uncommon. On the other hand, take the case of a teenage girl with a history of continuous nasal congestion since birth. Suppose her nose clears up within three days of removing all dairy products from her diet. Furthermore, every time she consumes dairy products in any form, even as an unsuspected ingredient in a casserole, her congestion comes right back. That is a good anecdote. The files of every good medical nutritionist are filled with such provocative tales. The medical orthodoxy can no longer use the "double-blind" argument as an excuse to keep its mind closed.

Fortunately, there are signs that things are beginning to change. More physicians than ever are discovering that there is more to the practice of medicine than what they learned in medical school. Eventually, because wisdom, economics and humanism demand it, nutritional therapy will replace certain aspects of current medical care. An alternative that is often safer, less expensive and more effective cannot remain on the fringes forever. One purpose I have in writing this book is to try to nudge medical care further in the direction that it must eventually go.

The other purpose of this book is to make you, the reader, aware of just how hazardous modern living can be to our health. Our toxic environment represents more than just a vague threat that we will all develop cancer sometime in the future. The facts seem to indicate that antimetabolites are making some of us ill already. It's encouraging to know that we can minimize some of the effects of our environment by increasing our vitamin B_6 intake. On the other hand, we must realize that vitamin therapy is only a stopgap measure in our struggle to preserve this polluted civilization. If present trends continue, our folly will eventually cripple the human race and destroy much of what is beautiful and sacred around us.

The story of vitamin B_6 is more than just a recital of biochemical theories and items of medical interest. It's a warning that, unless we stem the tide, antimetabolites and other toxins will ultimately get the best of us. While it's gratifying and exciting to see the good that vitamin therapy can do, it's also frightening to realize that so many people need scores or even hundreds of times as much vitamin B_6 as their ancestors did.

What You Can Do

What can you do to help reduce the potential danger of antimetabolites? On a personal level, you can take steps to avoid, whenever reasonably possible, exposure to suspected toxins. Many of the compounds that interfere with B_6 are in the food supply, so your diet is a good place to start. Do your best to avoid foods fried in vegetable oil that has been heated for prolonged periods, since heated vegetable oils are easily converted to peroxides and other toxic substances. It's especially wise to avoid the lowly potato chip. At one time, their salt content alone was enough to put potato chips on the "not recommended" list. Considering that this common snack is drenched in an oil that causes vitamin B₆ deficiency in rats, and considering that they may contain up to 160 parts per million of maleic hydrazide (a suspected B₆ antagonist), potato chips are not one of your healthier snacks.

Foods and drugs containing tartrazine (FD&C Yellow No. 5) should also be left alone when possible. The body converts this widely used food dye into a compound that probably inhibits B₆ metabolism. Heavily processed foods and foods with caramel color added may also contain B₆ antagonists and so should be avoided. If you smoke, try to quit; and if you don't smoke, don't start. Tobacco is a source of both hydrazine and maleic hydrazide. You might also consider reducing your intake of button mushrooms since they contain *agaritine,* an antimetabolite of vitamin B₆.

If you're able to locate fruits and vegetables that haven't been treated with pesticides, herbicides, fungicides, ripening agents or sprout inhibitors, then by all means use them. Some of these chemicals are hydrazine or hydrazide compounds and are suspected vitamin B₆ antagonists. Unfortunately, untreated produce is difficult to find in many parts of the country. If necessary, take matters into your own hands. Dig a large garden in your backyard and learn the techniques of organic gardening. Build your own greenhouse and reap the benefits of hydrazine-free winters. Let your grocer know why you no longer buy his produce.

Donate money to organizations that are doing scientific research in the public interest. Make it clear to traditional research institutions that you'll no longer support them unless they begin looking at new approaches. Urge your representative in Washington to support funding for research into nutrition and environmental pollution. We can no longer allow the funding of medical research to come from organizations that have a vested interest in deciding which questions will be asked (or avoided). As long as scientists remain dependent on the tobacco, food-processing and chemical industries for grant money, they'll be less likely to jeopardize their funding by asking the "wrong" questions. For scientific research to serve the public interest, funding must be available from the public sector or from private foundations that are truly dedicated to the public welfare.

With more research, it will become more obvious to everyone just what our environment and our diet are doing to us. As we become better informed, the path we must take will become clearer. We have an uphill battle ahead of us to regain our health and to ensure that this planet will support life far into the future.

B_6's 22
Biochemistry in Action

Vitamin B_6 is one of the most versatile nutrients. It plays a role in crucial biochemical reactions in every organ and every cell in our body. This chapter is a biochemistry lesson to show how B_6 works. Although the material is somewhat technical, it provides a background so you can better understand and appreciate the clinical uses of this vitamin. Although the biochemical functions of B_6 are quite fascinating, it's not necessary for you to learn all the details in this chapter to understand the rest of the information in the book.

Three Natural Forms

Vitamin B_6 occurs in three different forms in nature: pyridoxine, pyridoxal and pyridoxamine. This group of substances is collectively called vitamin B_6. Chemically, these compounds are interchangeable, and they are all equally effective in curing vitamin B_6 deficiency. Pyridoxine is the form of vitamin B_6 that is found in supplements and used most frequently in nutrition experiments; consequently, the entire group of vitamin B_6 compounds is often called "pyridoxine."

B_6 must first be converted to its active form—called pyridoxal phosphate (PLP)—to perform its functions in the body. This conversion takes place only if adequate amounts of riboflavin (vitamin B_2) are present.[1] This means that a riboflavin deficiency can impair vitamin B$_6$'s ability to do its job. Some people have difficulty converting pyridoxine to PLP because of an unknown biochemical defect, so pyridoxine supplements may not do them much good, even if their problems are caused by vitamin B$_6$ deficiency. Scientists have found that PLP injections help some of these people, but the research is still in its infancy.

Recently, oral supplements of PLP have appeared on the market. Studies in animals indicate that when this form of B$_6$ is taken by mouth, it is largely broken down in the gastrointestinal tract and only a small percentage is absorbed intact.[2] Although very little research has been done so far, some medical nutritionists feel that PLP supplements are beneficial in selected cases where pyridoxine doesn't work well.

Enzyme Actions

Most of B$_6$'s activities are a direct result of a single function: It is a cofactor to enzyme systems. An enzyme is a protein molecule that facilitates biochemical reactions. For example, when glutamic acid (an amino acid) dissolves in a glass of water, the laws of equilibrium dictate that a certain percentage will eventually be converted into another molecule, called GABA (gamma-aminobutyric acid). But this conversion could take a long time to occur, possibly hundreds or even thousands of years, if it weren't for enzyme action. GABA, which plays an important role in brain function, is produced solely from glutamic acid. If we had to sit around for years, waiting for a few glutamic acid molecules to be converted randomly into GABA, our brains would cease to function. Enzymes speed up reactions like this one that were going to occur anyway.

Nearly every biological function in our body is aided by enzymes. Scientists have discovered hundreds of enzymes, responsible for thousands of different biochemical tasks. Most of these enzymes require a helper, usually a vitamin or mineral, called a coenzyme or cofactor. Without the necessary cofactor, the enzyme couldn't do its job and important reactions would never take place.

Vitamin B$_6$ is the cofactor for more than 50 different enzymes. If the body lacks an adequate supply of this vitamin, or if it's unable to use its supply, the body chemistry could break down in any number of ways. Here are some of the key biochemical reactions vitamin B$_6$ participates in.

Vitamin B_6 is the coenzyme for a series of enzymes, called transaminases, that work in protein metabolism. These enzymes transfer ammonia molecules from one amino acid (protein building block) to another. Protein metabolism depends on constant transamination, as one amino acid is destroyed and another is created. Without normal protein synthesis, there would be no enzymes, no insulin and no antibodies; life itself would be impossible.

Vitamin B_6 plays a role in energy metabolism, too. One of the B_6-dependent enzymes, glycogen phosphorylase, converts stored carbohydrate into sugars to be used for fuel.

Vitamin B_6 is also involved in metabolizing essential fatty acids, notably linoleic and linolenic acids, which must be present in the diet to ensure normal health. When animals are fed a diet deficient in these essential fatty acids, they lose weight, develop skin problems and eventually die. These effects can be delayed or prevented by increasing the amount of B_6 in the diet. Conversely, supplements of essential fatty acids can delay the damage caused by a B_6-deficient diet.

David F. Horrobin, M.D., Ph.D., an authority on essential fatty acids, believes that these nutrients interact through a group of compounds known as prostaglandins, hormonelike substances that exert a wide range of effects on the heart, blood vessels, brain, kidneys, reproductive system, immune system and other tissues. Prostaglandins are made from the essential fatty acids. One of the prostaglandins that appears to be particularly important is called prostaglandin E1 (PGE1). A growing body of evidence suggests that deficiency of PGE1 is related to schizophrenia, hyperactivity, heart disease, cancer and the so-called autoimmune diseases.[3] Apparently, vitamin B_6 is required to convert linoleic acid into PGE1 (Fig. 1). If so, B_6 deficiency could play a role in any of the diseases related to PGE1.

Vitamin B_6 is the cofactor for another enzyme, called lysyl oxidase,[4] which is needed to strengthen the connective tissue in our body. Long protein fibers, such as collagen and elastin, provide structural support for the various tissues that make up our body. These fibers, which lie side by side, must somehow be joined together to resist pulling and tearing. Lysyl oxidase causes certain amino acids on one fiber to form a bond with amino acids on the adjacent chain. In a sense, this B_6-dependent enzyme weaves a cloth out of a series of threads. Without adequate vitamin B_6, lysyl oxidase would not function properly, and the connective tissue would lack tensile strength. Since weakness of the connective tissue of arteries may be a major cause of atherosclerosis

Figure 1. B₆'s Role in Forming PGE1

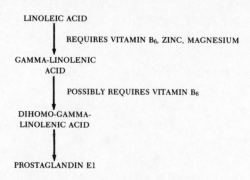

SOURCE: *Journal of Holistic Medicine,* vol. 3, no. 2, 1981, p. 118.

(hardening of the arteries), vitamin B_6 may help prevent the modern epidemic of cardiovascular disease.

Vitamin B_6 also plays a crucial role in metabolizing the amino acid tryptophan. This essential amino acid is the focal point of an interesting and complex biochemical system that affects human health in a number of ways. Tryptophan metabolism can proceed in several directions, giving rise to a range of metabolites (by-products) (see Fig. 2). The availability of vitamin B_6 determines in part which by-products of tryptophan will be produced. Some of these metabolites perform functions that are likely to affect human health and disease.

Serotonin is one such substance. This compound is found in the brain, where it functions as a neurotransmitter (chemical messenger). The conversion of tryptophan to serotonin requires vitamin B_6 and is impaired when not enough of this vitamin is present. Serotonin deficiency has been linked to depression, hyperactivity and other psychiatric problems. As we have seen, the need for additional B_6 appears to be a contributing factor in various emotional disorders. Some hyperactive and depressed people with low serotonin levels have noted dramatic improvements in their symptoms after treatment with large doses of vitamin B_6.

Niacinamide is also synthesized from tryptophan in a series of steps that require B_6. Without an adequate supply of B_6, we could become deficient in niacinamide as well. Of course, niacinamide occurs naturally in food, although typical processed American food contains very little. For people who subsist on such a diet, production from tryptophan would be an important secondary source of niacinamide.

Figure 2. B₆'s Role in Tryptophan Metabolism

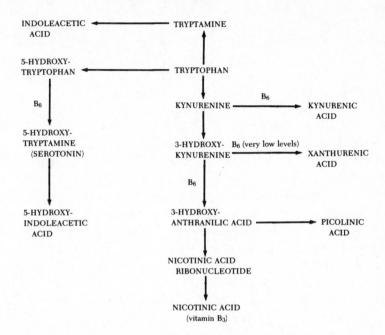

SOURCE: Winston, Frank. "Oral Contraceptives, Pyridoxine, and Depression." *American Journal of Psychiatry*, November, 1973, p. 138.

Another metabolite of tryptophan related to vitamin B₆ is called picolinic acid. This interesting compound is produced from tryptophan in a series of steps that require vitamin B₆. Picolinic acid appears to increase the effectiveness of zinc, an essential trace mineral. Zinc has recently been receiving a great deal of attention as a remedy for acne, skin ulcers, boils, stomach ulcers, psychiatric disorders, sexual dysfunction and a host of other ailments, though in many cases the results are not entirely satisfactory, even with very large doses. Part of the problem is getting zinc to places in the body where it's needed. In some cases, zinc is not well absorbed from the intestinal tract or transported adequately into the cells. Picolinic acid appears to bind to zinc and transport it to exactly the right places.[5,6] A colleague who is studying zinc picolinate (the zinc salt of picolinic acid) has found it to be more effective at a much smaller dose than other forms of zinc (such as gluconate, orotate or amino acid-chelated). Zinc picolinate is not commercially available right now, but picolinic acid can be produced by the body from tryptophan if adequate amounts of vitamin B₆ are present.

On the other hand, if B$_6$ is lacking, not enough picolinic acid can be produced, and zinc absorption can be impaired.

There is also evidence that picolinic acid helps prevent cancer. In one experiment, mice injected with tumor cells were also given injections of picolinic acid. Compared with animals that did not receive the picolinic acid, these mice had smaller tumors and lived longer.[7] If picolinic acid helps prevent cancer, and vitamin B$_6$ promotes synthesis of picolinic acid, B$_6$ might also be important in preventing cancer.

Xanthurenic acid is another by-product of tryptophan metabolism produced when the body lacks vitamin B$_6$. In fact, the presence of xanthurenic acid in the urine (as measured by the tryptophan load test explained in chapter 1) is one criterion used to diagnose B$_6$ deficiency. Xanthurenic acid has the unusual property of being able to bind to insulin and render it inactive. This action of xanthurenic acid could have important consequences, since inactivation of insulin could lead to diabetes. Injection of xanthurenic acid into animals has indeed produced diabetes. Furthermore, diabetics often have excessive xanthurenic acid. Since vitamin B$_6$ supplements usually prevent tryptophan from being converted to this harmful metabolite, B$_6$ might help prevent diabetes. There is also evidence that xanthurenic acid could promote (and vitamin B$_6$ could prevent) bladder cancer (see chapter 8).

Another biochemical reaction that requires B$_6$ is the conversion of the amino acid tyrosine to norepinephrine. Like serotonin, norepinephrine is a neurotransmitter that appears to play a role in mental depression. Some depressed people have low levels of norepinephrine in their brain. Vitamin B$_6$ may help relieve depression in certain cases by raising the level of this important neurotransmitter.

On its way to becoming norepinephrine, tyrosine must first be converted to dopamine, another compound with important functions in the nervous system. A deficiency of dopamine in the brain is associated with Parkinson's disease, a severe neurological disorder. The relationship among vitamin B$_6$, dopamine and Parkinson's disease is rather complicated, and was discussed more fully in chapter 19.

Vitamin B$_6$ is a cofactor for the enzyme that converts the amino acid glutamic acid into the neurotransmitter GABA. This neurotransmitter inhibits rather than stimulates brain activity. There is a theory that a deficiency of this inhibitor molecule may be one cause of epileptic seizures. Although this theory has not been proved, vitamin B$_6$ is known to prevent seizures in some epileptics.

Vitamins E and B$_6$ also seem to be interrelated. In one study, rats were fed a diet low in both these vitamins. This diet caused a rise in the urinary excretion of creatine, indicating that muscle damage was occurring. This rise in urinary creatine could be prevented by supplementing the diet either with vitamin E or with B_6. This study suggested that vitamin E can partly compensate for a deficiency of B_6, and vice versa.[8]

Magnesium is probably vitamin B_6's most important partner. Throughout this book there are numerous examples of how these nutrients work together to prevent and treat disease. Magnesium and B_6 are frequently found as cofactors for the same enzymes.[9] Without vitamin B_6, magnesium apparently has difficulty traveling into cells, where it performs most of its functions. In one study, doctors measured the concentration of magnesium in the blood plasma and red blood cells of nine women. Three of these women had low levels in the plasma, and all had low red blood cell concentrations of magnesium. Each of the women was then given vitamin B_6, 100 milligrams twice a day for four weeks. After taking B_6, plasma levels of magnesium increased and red blood cell levels doubled. The results of this study suggested that vitamin B_6 plays a role in the transport of magnesium into cells.[10] In the clinic, treatment with magnesium and B_6 together is often more effective than either of these nutrients alone. The combination of magnesium and B_6 appears to be beneficial in some cases of heart disease, diabetes, kidney stones and certain psychiatric problems.

Nutritional biochemistry is quite complicated and often poorly understood. A few of the reactions discussed in this chapter are considerably more involved than this brief overview has indicated, but I've simplified them to show you how important vitamin B_6 is for human health. I've omitted others that were discussed at length in earlier chapters.

By now I hope that it's obvious that vitamin B_6 plays a key role in the workings of the body. Because of its versatility, deficiency of B_6 could conceivably cause any number of different symptoms and illnesses. That's what this book is about.

Notes

Chapter 1: How Much Do We Need?

1. "Vitamin C and Infection." *Lancet*, July 22, 1944, p. 118.

2. Hansen, Arild E. "Serum Lipid Changes and Therapeutic Effects of Various Oils in Infantile Eczema." *Proceedings of the Society for Experimental Biology and Medicine*, November, 1933, pp. 160–161.

3. Kuh, Clifford. "A Study of Vitamin A in Relation to Experimental Cancer." *Yale Journal of Biology and Medicine*, vol. 5, no. 123, 1932, pp. 150–152.

4. Phalen, George S. "Reflections on 21 Years' Experience with the Carpal-Tunnel Syndrome." *Journal of the American Medical Association*, May 25, 1970, pp. 1365–1367.

5. Ettinger, Bruce. "Calcium Oxalate Stones: A Reappraisal of Their Work-Up and Prevention." *Medical Times*, November, 1981, pp. 20s–28s.

6. Kirksey, Avanelle et al. "Vitamin B_6 Nutritional Status of a Group of Female Adolescents." *American Journal of Clinical Nutrition*, June, 1978, pp. 946–954.

7. Buffoni, F.; Ignesti, G.; and Pirisino, R. "3-Hydrazinopyridazine Derivatives as Inhibitors of the Copper Containing Amine Oxidases." *Farmaco* [*Edizione Scientifica*], June, 1977, pp. 404–413.

8. Buffoni, F. et al. "3-Hydrazinopyridazine Derivatives in Inhibitors of Pyridoxal-Phosphate Dependent Enzymes." *Farmaco* [*Edizione Scientifica*], October, 1980, pp. 848–855.

9. Toth, Bela, and Erickson, James. "Reversal of the Toxicity of Hydrazine Analogues by Pyridoxine Hydrochloride." *Toxicology*, February, 1977, pp. 31–36.

10. Kirklin, James K. et al. "Treatment of Hydrazine-Induced Coma with Pyridoxine." *New England Journal of Medicine*, April 22, 1976, pp. 938–939.

11. MacNaughton, Michael G.; Stauffer, Thomas B.; and Stone, Daniel A. "Environmental Chemistry and Management of Hydrazine." *Aviation, Space, and Environmental Medicine*, March, 1981, pp. 149–153.

12. Toth, Bela. "Synthetic and Naturally Occurring Hydrazines as Possible Cancer Causative Agents." *Cancer Research*, December, 1975, pp. 3693–3697.

13. Roepke, Judith B., and Kirksey, Avanelle. "Effect of Smoking and Vitamin B_6 Supplementation during Pregnancy on Maternal Vitamin B_6 Status and Infant Birth Weight." *Federation Proceedings*, March 5, 1983, p. 1066.

14. Biehl, J. P., and Vilter, Richard W. "Effects of Isoniazid on Pyridoxine Metabolism." *Journal of the American Medical Association*, December 25, 1954, pp. 1549–1552.

15. Snider, Dixie E., Jr. "Pyridoxine Supplementation during Isoniazid Therapy." *Tubercle*, vol. 61, no. 4, 1980, pp. 191–196.

16. Sievers, Maurice L. et al. "Treatment of Isoniazid Overdose." *Journal of the American Medical Association*, February 5, 1982, pp. 583–584.

17. Rumsby, P. C., and Shepherd, D. M. "Effect of Penicillamine, Hydrallazine, and Phenelzine on the Function of Pyridoxal-5'-Phosphate." *British Journal of Pharmacology*, July, 1979, p. 453P–454P.

18. Kirkendall, Walter M., and Page, Elisabeth B. "Polyneuritis Occurring during Hydralazine Therapy: Report of Two Cases and Discussion of Adverse Reactions to Hydralazine." *Journal of the American Medical Association*, May 24, 1958, pp. 427–432.

19. Toth, B. "Actual New Cancer-Causing Hydrazines, Hydrazides, and Hydrazones." *Journal of Cancer Research and Clinical Oncology*, vol. 97, no. 2, 1980, pp. 97–108.

20. Dunleavy, D. L. "Phenelzine and Edema." *British Medical Journal*, May 21, 1977, p. 1353.

21. Newsome, William H. "Residues of Maleic Hydrazide in Field-Treated Potatoes." *Journal of Agricultural and Food Chemistry*, November-December, 1980, pp. 1312–1313.

22. Senter, S. D.; Lyon, B. G.; and Horton, B. D. "A Research Note: Effects of Different Concentrations of Succinic Acid-2,2-Dimethylhydrazide on the Flavor of Puree from Fresh and Canned Freestone Peaches." *Journal of Food Science*, vol. 40, no. 5, 1975, pp. 1103–1104.

23. Lee, Mary et al. "Tartrazine-Containing Drugs." *Drug Intelligence and Clinical Pharmacy*, October, 1981, pp. 782–788.

24. Zlotlow, Mark J., and Settipane, Guy A. "Allergic Potential of Food Additives: A Report of a Case of Tartrazine Sensitivity without Aspirin Intolerance." *American Journal of Clinical Nutrition*, July, 1977, pp. 1023–1025.

25. Ryan, A. J.; Welling, P. G.; and (the late) Wright, S. E. "Further Studies on the Metabolism of Tartrazine and Related Compounds in the Intact Rat." *Food and Cosmetics Toxicology*, vol. 7, no. 4, July, 1969, pp. 287–294.

26. Prasad, Ananda S. et al. "Effect of Oral Contraceptives on Nutrients: III. Vitamins B_6, B_{12}, and Folic Acid." *American Journal of Obstetrics and Gynecology*, August 15, 1976, pp. 1063–1069.

27. Rothschild, Bruce. "Pyridoxine Deficiency." *Archives of Internal Medicine*, April, 1982, p. 840.

28. Cohen, Archibald C. "Pyridoxine in the Prevention and Treatment of Convulsions and Neurotoxicity Due to Cycloserine." *Annals of the New York Academy of Sciences*, September 30, 1969, pp. 346–349.

29. Roepke, Judith L., and Kirksey, Avanelle. "Vitamin B_6 Nurtiture during Pregnancy and Lactation: II. The Effect of Long-Term Use of Oral Contraceptives." *American Journal of Clinical Nutrition*, November, 1979, pp. 2257–2264.

30. Wickizer, Thomas M. et al. "Polychlorinated Biphenyl Contamination of Nursing Mothers' Milk in Michigan." *American Journal of Public Health*, February, 1981, pp. 132–137.

31. Chang, King-Jen et al. "Immunologic Evaluation of Patients with Polychlorinated Biphenyl Poisoning: Determination of Lymphocyte Subpopulations." *Toxicology and Applied Pharmacology*, October, 1981, pp. 58–63.

32. Mes, Jos; Davies, David J; and Turton, Davida. "Polychlorinated Biphenyl and Other Chlorinated Hydrocarbon Residues in Adipose Tissue of Canadians." *Bulletin of Environmental Contamination and Toxicology*, January, 1982, pp. 97–104.

33. Fujiwara, Mayuki, and Kuriyama, Kinya. "Effect of PCB (Polychlorobiphenyls) on L-Ascorbic Acid, Pyridoxal Phosphate and Riboflavin Contents in Various Organs and on Hepatic Metabolism of L-Ascorbic Acid in the Rat." *Japanese Journal of Pharmacology*, October, 1977, pp. 621–627.

34. Witting, Lloyd A. et al. "The Relationship of Pyridoxine and Riboflavin to the Nutritional Value of Polymerized Fats." *Journal of the American Oil Chemists' Society*, September, 1957, pp. 421–424.

35. Spector, Reynold, and Huntoon, Sheryl. "Effects of Caramel Color (Ammonia Process) on Mammalian Vitamin B_6 Metabolism." *Toxicology and Applied Pharmacology*, January, 1982, pp. 172–178.

36. Gregory, Jesse F., III. "Effects of Epsilon-Pyridoxyllysine Bound to Dietary Protein on the Vitamin B_6 Status of Rats." *Journal of Nutrition*, May, 1980, pp. 995–1005.

37. Klosterman, H. J.; Lamoureux, G. L.; and Parsons, J. L. "Isolation, Characterization, and Synthesis of Linatine. A Vitamin B_6 Antagonist from Flaxseed *(Linum usitatissimum)*." *Biochemistry*, January, 1967, pp. 170–177.

38. Klosterman, Harold J. "Vitamin B_6 Antagonists of Natural Origin." *Journal of Agricultural and Food Chemistry*, vol. 22, no. 1, 1974, pp. 13–16.

39. Malinow, M. R. et al. "Systemic Lupus Erythematosus-Like Syndrome in Monkeys Fed Alfalfa Sprouts: Role of Nonprotein Amino Acid." *Science*, April, 1982, pp. 415–417.

40. National Research Council. "Recommended Dietary Allowances—Definition and Applications." In *Recommended Dietary Allowances*. 9th ed. National Academy of Sciences, 1980, p. 1.

41. Williams, Roger J. "A New Hope for Better Health." In *Nutrition Against Disease: Environmental Prevention*, Pitman Publishing, 1971, pp. 37–50.

42. Frimpter, George W.; Andelman, Robert J.; and George, Walter F. "Vitamin B_6-Dependency Syndromes: New Horizons in Nutrition." *American Journal of Clinical Nutrition*, June 1969, pp. 794–805.

43. Sauberlich, H. E. et al. "Biochemical Assessment of the Nutritional Status of Vitamin B_6 in the Human." *American Journal of Clinical Nutrition*, June, 1972, pp. 629–642.

44. Azuma, Junichi et al. "Apparent Deficiency of Vitamin B$_6$ in Typical Individuals Who Commonly Serve as Normal Controls." *Research Communications in Chemical Pathology and Pharmacology*, June, 1976, pp. 343–348.

Chapter 2: The Premenstrual Syndrome

1. Armitage, Karen J.; Schneiderman, Lawrence, J.; and Bass, Robert A. "Response of Physicians to Medical Complaints in Men and Women." *Journal of the American Medical Association*, May 18, 1979, pp. 2186–2187.

2. Reid, Robert L., and Yen, S. S. C. "Premenstrual Syndrome." *American Journal of Obstetrics and Gynecology*, vol. 139, no. 1, 1981, pp. 85–104.

3. Lauersen, Neils H., and Graves, Zoe R. "A New Approach to Premenstrual Syndrome." *The Female Patient*, April, 1983, pp. 41–55.

4. Mattsson, B., and von Schoultz, B. "A Comparison Between Lithium, Placebo and a Diuretic in Premenstrual Tension." *Acta Psychiatrica Scandinavica*, Suppl. 255, 1974, pp. 75–84.

5. MacGregor, G. A. et al. "Is 'Idiopathic' Edema Idiopathic?" *Lancet*, February 24, 1979, pp. 397–400.

6. Adams, P. W. et al. "Influence of Oral Contraceptives, Pyridoxine (Vitamin B$_6$), and Tryptophan on Carbohydrate Metabolism." *Lancet*, April 10, 1976, pp. 759–764.

7. McIntosh, E. N. "Treatment of Women with the Galactorrhea-Amenorrhea Syndrome with Pyridoxine (Vitamin B$_6$)." *Journal of Clinical Endocrinology and Metabolism*, vol. 42, no. 6, 1976, pp. 1192–1195.

8. Adams, P. W. et al. "Effect of Pyridoxine Hydrochloride (Vitamin B$_6$) upon Depression Associated with Oral Contraception." *Lancet*, April 28, 1973, pp. 897–904.

9. Nelson, Marjorie M.; Lyons, William R.; and Evans, Herbert M. "Maintenance of Pregnancy in Pyridoxine-Deficient Rats When Injected with Estrone and Progesterone." *Endocrinology*, June, 1951, pp. 726–732.

10. Cotzias, George C., and Papavasilou, Paul S. "Blocking the Negative Effects of Pyridoxine on Patients Receiving Levodopa." *Journal of the American Medical Association*, March 1, 1971, pp. 1504–1505.

11. Bhagavan, Hemmige N.; Coleman, Mary; and Coursin, David. "The Effect of Pyridoxine Hydrochloride on Blood Serotonin and Pyridoxal Phosphate Contents in Hyperactive Children." *Pediatrics*, March, 1975, pp. 437–441.

12. Abraham, Guy E., and Hargrove, Joel T. "Effect of Vitamin B₆ on Premenstrual Symptomatology in Women with Premenstrual Tension Syndrome. A Double-Blind Crossover Study." *Infertility*, vol. 3, no. 2, 1980, pp. 155–165.

13. Biskind, Morton S.; Biskind, Gerson R.; and Biskind, Leonard H. "Nutritional Deficiency in the Etiology of Menorrhagia, Metrorrhagia, Cystic Mastitis, and Premenstrual Tension." *Surgery, Gynecology and Obstetrics*, January, 1944, pp. 49–57.

14. Zondek, Bernhard, and Brzezinski, Aron. "Inactivation of Oestrogenic Hormone by Women with Vitamin B Deficiency." *Journal of Obstetrics and Gynaecology of the British Commonwealth*, June, 1948, pp. 273–280.

15. Leklem, J. E. et al. "Metabolism of Tryptophan and Niacin in Oral Contraceptive Users Receiving Controlled Intakes of Vitamin B₆." *American Journal of Clinical Nutrition*, February, 1975, pp. 146–156.

16. Kerr, G. D. "The Management of the Premenstrual Syndrome." *Current Medical Research and Opinion*, vol. 4, suppl. 4, 1977, pp. 29–34.

17. Snider, B. Leonard, and Dieteman, David F. "Pyridoxine Therapy for Premenstrual Acne Flare." *Archives of Dermatology*, July, 1974, pp. 130–131.

18. Rimland, Bernard; Callaway, Enoch; and Dreyfus, Pierre. "The Effect of High Doses of Vitamin B₆ on Autistic Children: A Double-Blind Crossover Study." *American Journal of Psychiatry*, April, 1978, pp. 472–475.

19. Debrovner, Charles H. "Premenstrual Syndrome." *Medical Aspects of Human Sexuality*, April, 1983, pp. 215–226.

Chapter 3: Pregnancy

1. National Research Council. "Trace Elements." In *Recommended Dietary Allowances*. 9th ed. National Academy of Sciences, 1980, p. 138.

2. Schuster, Karen; Bailey, Lynn B.; and Mahan, Charles S. "Vitamin B₆ Status of Low-Income Adolescent and Adult Pregnant Women and the Condition of Their Infants at Birth." *American Journal of Clinical Nutrition*, September, 1981, pp. 1731–1735.

3. Kirksey, Avanelle et al. "Vitamin B₆ Nutritional Status of a Group of Female Adolescents." *American Journal of Clinical Nutrition*, June, 1978, pp. 946–954.

4. Wachstein, M., and Gudaitis, A. "Disturbance of Vitamin B₆ Metabolism in Pregnancy." *Journal of Laboratory and Clinical Medicine*, October, 1952, pp. 550–557.

5. Wachstein, M., and Gudaitis, M. T. "Disturbance of Vitamin B₆ Metabolism in Pregnancy." *American Journal of Obstetrics and Gynecology*, December, 1953, pp. 1207–1213.

6. Coursin, David B., and Brown, Virginia C. "Changes in Vitamin B₆ during Pregnancy." *American Journal of Obstetrics and Gynecology*, December, 1961, pp. 1307–1311.

7. Reinken, L., and Dapunt, O. "Vitamin B₆ Nutriture during Pregnancy." *International Journal of Vitamin and Nutrition Research*, vol. 48, no. 4, 1978, pp. 341–347.

8. Bapurao, S.; Raman, Leela; and Tulpule, P. G. "Biochemical Assessment of Vitamin B₆ Nutritional Status in Pregnant Women with Orolingual Manifestations." *American Journal of Clinical Nutrition*, October, 1982, pp. 581–586.

9. National Research Council. "Water Soluble Vitamins: Vitamin B₆." In *Recommended Dietary Allowances*. 9th ed. National Academy of Sciences, 1980, pp. 96–106.

10. Hillman, Robert W. et al. "Pyridoxine Supplementation during Pregnancy: Clinical and Laboratory Observations." *American Journal of Clinical Nutrition*, June, 1963, pp. 427–430.

11. Hillman, Robert W.; Cabaud, Philip G.; and Schenone, Roger A. "The Effects of Pyridoxine Supplements on the Dental Caries Experience of Pregnant Women." *American Journal of Clinical Nutrition*, June, 1962, pp. 512–515.

12. Brent, Robert L. "The Bendectin Saga: Another American Tragedy." *Teratology*, April, 1983, pp. 283–286.

13. Willis, Raymond S. et al. "Clinical Observation in Treatment of Nausea and Vomiting in Pregnancy with Vitamins B$_1$ and B$_6$." *American Journal of Obstetrics and Gynecology*, August, 1942, pp. 265–271.

14. Silbernagel, Wynne M., and Burt, Olan P. "Effects of Pyridoxine on Nausea and Vomiting of Pregnancy." *Ohio State Medical Journal*, December, 1943, pp. 1113–1114.

15. Weinstein, B. Bernard et al. "Oral Administration of Pyridoxine Hydrochloride in the Treatment of Nausea and Vomiting of Pregnancy." *American Journal of Obstetrics and Gynecology*, March, 1944, pp. 389–394.

16. Gant, Von H. et al. "Vitamin B$_6$ Depletion in Women with Hyperemesis Gravidarum." *Wiener Klinische Wochenschrift*, September 5, 1975, p. 510.

17. Hesseltine, H. Close. "Pyridoxine Failure in Nausea and Vomiting of Pregnancy." *American Journal of Obstetrics and Gynecology*, January, 1946, pp. 82–86.

18. AMA Department of Drugs. "Antiemetics." In *AMA Drug Evaluations*. 3d ed. PSG Publishing Company, 1977, p. 1091.

19. Goodhart, Robert S., and Shils, Maurice E., eds. "The Vitamins." In *Modern Nutrition in Health and Disease*. Lea and Febiger, 1980, p. 225.

20. Baum, G. et al. "Meclizine and Pyridoxine in Pregnancy Sickness." *Practitioner*, 1963, pp. 251–253.

21. Klieger, Jack A. et al. "Abnormal Pyridoxine Metabolism in Toxemia of Pregnancy." *Annals of the New York Academy of Sciences*, September 30, 1969, pp. 288–296.

22. Wachstein, M., and Graffeo, Louis W. "Influence of Vitamin B$_6$ on the Incidence of Preeclampsia." *Obstetrics and Gynecology*, August, 1956, pp. 177–180.

23. Ellis, John M., and Presley, James. *Vitamin B$_6$: The Doctor's Report*. Harper and Row, 1973, pp. 90–113.

24. Hammar, Mats; Larsson, Lasse; and Tegler, Lennart. "Calcium Treatment of Leg Cramps in Pregnancy." *Acta Obstetricia et Gynecologica Scandinavica*, vol. 60, no. 4, 1981, pp. 345–347.

25. Hambridge, K. M. "Zinc Nutritional Status during Pregnancy: A Longitudinal Study." *American Journal of Clinical Nutrition*, March, 1983, pp. 429–442.

26. Caddell, Joan L.; Saier, Fulton L.; and Thomason, Carol A. "Parenteral Magnesium Load Tests in Postpartum American Women." *American Journal of Clinical Nutrition*, October, 1975, pp. 1099–1104.

27. Beach, Richard S.; Gershwin, M. Eric; and Hurley, Lucille S. "Gestational Zinc Deprivation in Mice: Persistence of Immunodeficiency for Three Generations." *Science*, October, 1982, pp. 469–471.

28. Singh, V. K.; Rohatgi, P.; and Sur, B. K. "A Study of Serum Magnesium in Various Types of Abortions." *Journal of Obstetrics and Gynaecology of India*, vol. 29, 1979, pp. 1174–1177.

29. Coelingh Bennink, H. J., and Schreurs, W. H. "Improvement of Oral Glucose Tolerance in Gestational Diabetes by Pyridoxine." *British Medical Journal*, July 5, 1975, pp. 13–15.

30. Spellacy, W. N.; Buhi, W. C.; and Birk, S. A. "Vitamin B_6 Treatment of Gestational Diabetes Mellitus." *American Journal of Obstetrics and Gynecology*, March 15, 1977, pp. 599–602.

31. Perkins, Richard P. "Failure of Pyridoxine to Improve Glucose Tolerance in Gestational Diabetes Mellitus." *Obstetrics and Gynecology*, September, 1977, pp. 370–372.

32. Gillmer, M. D., and Mazibuko, D. "Pyridoxine Treatment of Chemical Diabetes in Pregnancy." *American Journal of Obstetrics and Gynecology*, March 1, 1979, pp. 499–502.

33. Wasynczuk, Anne; Kirksey, Avanelle; and Morré, Dorothy M. "Effect of Maternal Vitamin B_6 Deficiency on Specific Regions of Developing Rat Brain: Amino Acid Metabolism." *Journal of Nutrition*, April, 1983, pp. 735–745.

34. Yoneda, Toshiyuki, and Pratt, Robert M. "Vitamin B_6 Reduces Cortisone-Induced Cleft Palate in the Mouse." *Teratology*, December, 1982, pp. 255–258.

35. Davis, Starkey D.; Nelson, Thomas; and Shepard, Thomas H. "Teratogenicity of Vitamin B_6 Deficiency: Omphalocele, Skeletal and Neural Defects, and Splenic Hypoplasia." *Science*, September, 1970, pp. 1329–1330.

36. Roepke, Judith L., and Kirksey, Avanelle. "Vitamin B$_6$ Nutriture during Pregnancy and Lactation." *American Journal of Clinical Nutrition*, November, 1979, pp. 2249–2256.

37. Brophy, Michael H., and Siiteri, Pentti K. "Pyridoxine Deficit in Toxemic Offspring with Potential Neurologic Correlations." *Neurology*, April, 1976, p. 363.

38. Roepke, Judith B., and Kirksey, Avanelle. "Effect of Smoking and Vitamin B$_6$ Supplementation during Pregnancy on Maternal Vitamin B$_6$ Status and Infant Birth Weight." *Federation Proceedings*, March 5, 1983, p. 1066.

39. Toth, Bela. "Synthetic and Naturally Occurring Hydrazines as Possible Cancer Causative Agents." *Cancer Research*, December, 1975, pp. 3693–3697.

40. Foukas, Matthias D. "An Antilactogenic Effect of Pyridoxine." *Journal of Obstetrics and Gynaecology of the British Commonwealth*, August, 1973, pp. 718–720.

41. Canales, E. S. et al. "The Influence of Pyridoxine on Prolactin Secretion and Milk Production in Women." *British Journal of Obstetrics and Gynaecology*, May, 1976, pp. 387–388.

Chapter 4: Depression

1. Teuting, Patricia; Koslow, Stephen H.; and Hirschfeld, Robert M. "Introduction." In *National Institute of Mental Health Science Reports: Special Report on Depression Research*. U.S. Department of Health and Human Services, 1981, p. 1.

2. Bureau of the Census. *Statistical Abstract of the United States 1982–83*. 103d ed. U.S. Government Printing Office, 1982, p. 81.

3. Maas, J. W. "Clinical and Biochemical Heterogeneity of Depressive Disorders." *Annals of Internal Medicine*, vol. 88, no. 4, 1978, pp. 556–563.

4. Pauling, Linus. "Orthomolecular Psychiatry." *Science*, April 19, 1968, pp. 265–271.

5. Lindberg, D. et al. "Symptom Reduction in Depression after Treatment with L-Tryptophan or Imipramine." *Acta Psychiatrica Scandinavica*, September, 1979, pp. 287–294.

6. Goldberg, Ivan K. "L-Tyrosine in Depression." *Lancet,* August 16, 1980, p. 364.

7. Green, A. R., and Curzon, G. "The Effect of Tryptophan Metabolites on Brain 5-Hydroxytryptamine Metabolism." *Biochemical Pharmacology,* June, 1970, pp. 2061–2068.

8. Adams, P. W. et al. "Effect of Pyridoxine Hydrochloride (Vitamin B$_6$) upon Depression Associated with Oral Contraception." *Lancet,* April 28, 1973, pp. 897–904.

9. Baumblatt, Michael J., and Winston, Frank. "Pyridoxine and the Pill." *Lancet,* April 18, 1970, pp. 832–833.

10. Russ, Carolyn S. et al. "Vitamin B$_6$ Status of Depressed and Obsessive-Compulsive Patients." *Nutrition Reports International,* April, 1983, pp. 867–873.

11. Nobbs, B. T. "Pyridoxal Phosphate Status in Clinical Depression." *Lancet,* March 9, 1974, pp. 405–406.

12. Pulkkinen, M. O.; Salminen, J.; and Virtanen, S. "Serum Vitamin B$_6$ in Pure Pregnancy Depression." *Acta Obstetricia et Gynecologica Scandinavica,* vol. 57, no. 5, 1978, pp. 471–472.

13. Livingston, J. E.; MacLeod, P. M.; and Applegarth, D. A. "Vitamin B$_6$ Status in Women with Postpartum Depression." *American Journal of Clinical Nutrition,* May, 1978, p. 886–891.

14. Daynes, G. "Cyanocobalamin in Postpartum Psychosis." *South African Medical Journal,* August 9, 1975, p. 1373.

15. Thornton, William E. "Folate Deficiency in Puerperal Psychosis." *American Journal of Obstetrics and Gynecology,* September 15, 1977, pp. 222–223.

16. Hallert, C.; Åström, J.; and Walan, A. "Reversal of Psychopathology in Adult Celiac Disease with the Aid of Pyridoxine (Vitamin B$_6$)." *Scandinavian Journal of Gastroenterology,* vol. 18, no. 2, 1983, p. 299.

17. Roepke, Judith B., and Kirksey, Avanelle. "Effect of Smoking and Vitamin B$_6$ Supplementation during Pregnancy on Maternal Vitamin B$_6$ Status and Infant Birth Weight." *Federation Proceedings,* March 5, 1983, p. 1066.

18. Chouinard, G. et al. "Tryptophan-Nicotinamide Combination in Depression." *Lancet,* January 29, 1977, p. 249.

Chapter 5: Hyperactivity

1. Cantwell, Dennis P. "Attention Deficit Disorders and Hyperactivity." *Medical Times*, February, 1982, pp. 42s–50s.

2. Silver, Larry B. "Minimal Brain Dysfunction: Understanding It and Treating It." *Resident & Staff Physician*, November, 1979, pp. 95–106.

3. *Physician's Desk Reference*. Medical Economics Company, 1983, p. 865.

4. Feingold, Ben F. "The K-P Diet." In *Why Your Child Is Hyperactive*. Random House, 1975, pp. 169–170.

5. "NIH Consensus Development Conference: Defined Diets and Childhood Hyperactivity." *Clinical Pediatrics*, October, 1982, pp. 627–630.

6. Prinz, Ronald J; Roberts, William A.; and Hantman, Elaine. "Dietary Correlates of Hyperactive Behavior in Children." *Journal of Consulting and Clinical Psychology*, vol. 48, no. 6, 1980, pp. 760–769.

7. Rapp, Doris J. "Food Allergy Treatment for Hyperkinesis." *Journal of Learning Disabilities*, vol. 12, no. 9, 1979, pp. 608–616.

8. Greenberg, Alan S., and Coleman, Mary. "Use of Blood Serotonin Levels for the Classification and Treatment of Hyperactive Behavior Disorders." *Neurology*, vol. 23, no. 428 (Abstract), 1973.

9. Coleman, Mary et al. "The Role of Whole Blood Serotonin Levels in Monitoring Vitamin B$_6$ and Drug Therapy in Hyperactive Children." *Agents and Actions*, vol. 5 (Abstract), 1975, p. 496.

10. Winston, Frank. "Oral Contraceptives, Pyridoxine and Depression." *American Journal of Psychiatry*, November, 1973, pp. 1217–1221.

11. Sauberlich, H. E. et al. "Biochemical Assessment of the Nutritional Status of Vitamin B$_6$ in the Human." *American Journal of Clinical Nutrition*, June, 1972, pp. 629–642.

12. Green, A. R., and Curzon, G. "The Effect of Tryptophan Metabolites on Brain 5-Hydroxytryptamine Metabolism." *Biochemical Pharmacology*, June, 1970, pp. 2061–2068.

13. Coleman, Mary et al. "A Preliminary Study of the Effect of Pyridoxine Administration in a Subgroup of Hyperkinetic Children: A

Double-Blind Crossover Comparison with Methylphenidate." *Biological Psychiatry*, vol. 14, no. 5, 1979, pp. 741–751.

14. Reed, James F., and Slaichert, William, "Statistical Proof in 'Negative' Trials." *Archives of Internal Medicine*, September, 1981, pp. 1307–1310.

15. Brenner, Arnold, and Wapnir, Paul A. "A Pyridoxine-Dependent Behavioral Disorder Unmasked by Isoniazid." *American Journal of Diseases of Children*, August, 1978, pp. 773–776.

16. Brenner, Arnold. Personal Communication.

17. Brenner, Arnold. "The Effects of Megadoses of Selected B Complex Vitamins on Children with Hyperkinesis: Controlled Studies with Long-Term Follow-up." *Journal of Learning Disabilities*, May, 1982, pp. 258–264.

18. Ryan, A. J.; Welling, P. G.; and (the late) Wright, S. E. "Further Studies on the Metabolism of Tartrazine and Related Compounds in the Intact Rat." *Food and Cosmetics Toxicology*, vol. 7, no. 4, July, 1969, pp. 287–294.

Chapter 6: Other Emotional Disorders

1. Heeley, A. F., and Roberts, G. E. "A Study of Tryptophan Metabolism in Psychotic Children." *Developmental Medicine and Child Neurology*, December 8, 1966, pp. 708–717.

2. Rimland, Bernard; Callaway, Enoch; and Dreyfus, Pierre. "The Effect of High Doses of Vitamin B$_6$ on Autistic Children: A Double-Blind Crossover Study." *American Journal of Psychiatry*, April, 1978, pp. 472–475.

3. Rimland, Bernard. "An Orthomolecular Study of Psychotic Chilren." *Journal of Orthomolecular Psychiatry*, vol. 3, no. 4, 1974, pp. 371–377.

4. Lelord, G. et al. "Effects of Pyridoxine and Magnesium on Autistic Symptoms—Initial Observations." *Journal of Autism and Developmental Disorders*, vol. 11, no. 2, 1981, pp. 219–230.

5. Abecasis, M. K. "Breath-holding Spells and Vitamin B$_6$." *Developmental Medicine and Child Neurology*, August, 1973, p. 541.

6. Pauling, Linus. "Orthomolecular Psychiatry." *Science*, April 19, 1968, pp. 265–271.

7. Pfeiffer, C. C. et al. "Treatment of Pyroluric Schizophrenia (Malvaria) with Large Doses of Pyridoxine and a Dietary Supplement of Zinc." *Journal of Orthomolecular Psychiatry*, vol. 3, no. 4, 1974, pp. 292–300.

8. Ananth, J. V.; Ban, T. A.; and Lehmann, H. E. "Potentiation of Therapeutic Effects of Nicotinic Acid by Pyridoxine in Chronic Schizophrenics." *Canadian Psychiatric Association Journal*, October, 1973, pp. 377–383.

9. DeVeaugh-Geiss, Joseph, and Manion, Lawrence. "High-Dose Pyridoxine in Tardive Dyskinesia." *Journal of Clinical Psychiatry*, June, 1978, pp. 573–575.

Chapter 7: Heart Disease

1. Goswami, A., and Sadhu, D. P. "Polyenoic Acid in Hypercholesterolemia Induced by Pyridoxine Deficiency in Rats." *Nature*, August 27, 1960, pp. 786–787.

2. Rose, G. A.; Thomson, W. B.; and Williams, R. T. "Corn Oil in Treatment of Ischaemic Heart Disease." *British Medical Journal*, June 12, 1965, pp. 1531–1533.

3. Malmros, Haqvin, "Diet, Lipids and Atherosclerosis." *Acta Medica Scandinavica*, vol. 207, no. 3, 1980, pp. 145–149.

4. Multiple Risk Factor Intervention Trial Research Group. "Multiple Risk Factor Intervention Trial: Risk Factor Changes and Mortality Results." *Journal of the American Medical Association*, vol. 248, no. 12, 1982, pp. 1465–1477.

5. Gaby, Alan R. "Nutritional Factors in Cardiovascular Disease." *Journal of Holistic Medicine*, vol. 5, no. 2, 1983, p. 815.

6. Taylor, C. B. et al. "Spontaneously Occurring Angiotoxic Derivatives of Cholesterol." *American Journal of Clinical Nutrition*, January, 1979, pp. 40–57.

7. Bird, Timothy A., and Levene, Charles I. "Lysyl Oxidase: Evidence that Pyridoxal Phosphate Is a Cofactor." *Biochemical and Biophysical Research Communications*, vol. 108, no. 3, 1982, pp. 1172–1180.

8. Levene C. I., and Murray, J. C. "The Aetiological Role of Maternal Vitamin B$_6$ Deficiency in the Development of Atherosclerosis." *Lancet*, March 19, 1977, pp. 628–629.

9. Rinehart, James F., and Greenberg, Louis D. "Vitamin B$_6$ Deficiency in the Rhesus Monkey." *American Journal of Clinical Nutrition*, vol. 4, no. 4, 1956, pp. 318–325.

10. Subbarao, K.; Kuchibhotia, J.; and Green, D. "Pyridoxine-Induced Inhibition of Platelet Aggregation and the Release Reaction." *Circulation*, vol. 56, no. 4, 1977, p. III–77.

11. "Is Vitamin B$_6$ an Antithrombotic Agent?" *Lancet*, June 13, 1981, pp. 1299–1300.

12. Packham, M.; Lam, S.; and Mustard, J. "Vitamin B$_6$ as an Antithrombotic Agent." *Lancet*, October 10, 1981, pp. 809–810.

13. Seronde, Joseph, Jr. "Cardiac Lesions and Related Findings in Young Vitamin B$_6$-Deficient Rats." *Journal of Nutrition*, vol. 72, 1960, pp. 53–65.

14. Mulvaney, D., and Seronde, J., Jr. "Electrocardiographic Changes in Vitamin B$_6$ Deficient Rats." *Cardiovascular Research*, September, 1979, pp. 506–513.

15. Ellis, John M., and Presley, James. *Vitamin B$_6$: The Doctor's Report*. Harper and Row, 1973.

Chapter 8: Cancer

1. American Cancer Society. *Cancer Facts and Figures*. American Cancer Society, 1984.

2. "Vitamin B$_6$ Deficiency and Immune Responses." *Nutrition Reviews*, June, 1976, pp. 188–189.

3. Chandra, R. K.; Au, B.; and Heresi, Gloria. "Single Nutrient Deficiency and Cell-Mediated Immune Responses: II. Pyridoxine." *Nutrition Research*, vol. 1, 1981, pp. 101–106.

4. Bryan, George T.; Brown, R. R.; and Price, J. M. "Mouse Bladder Carcinogenicity of Certain Tryptophan Metabolites and Other Aromatic Nitrogen Compounds Suspended in Cholesterol." *Cancer Research*, May, 1964, pp. 596–602.

5. Yoshida, Osamu; Brown, Raymond R.; and Bryan, George T. "Relationship Between Tryptophan Metabolism and Heterotopic Recurrences of Human Urinary Bladder Tumors." *Cancer*, April, 1970, pp. 773–780.

6. Byar, David, and Blackard, Clyde. "Comparisons of Placebo, Pyridoxine and Topical Thiotepa in Preventing Recurrence of Stage 1 Bladder Cancer." *Urology*, December, 1977, pp. 556–561.

7. Brown, R. R. et al. "Metabolism of Tryptophan in Patients with Bladder Cancer." *Acta Unio Internationalis Contra Cancrum*, vol. 16, 1960, pp. 299–303.

8. Miller, Carolyn T. et al. "Relative Importance of Risk Factors in Bladder Carcinogenesis." *Journal of Chronic Diseases*, January, 1978, pp. 51–56.

9. Williams, Harry L., and Wiegand, Ronald G. "Xanthurenic Acid Excretion and Possible Pyridoxine Deficiency Produced by Isonicotinic Acid Hydrazide and Other Convulsant Hydrazides." *Journal of Pharmacology and Experimental Therapeutics*, April, 1960, pp. 344–348.

10. Toth, Bela. "Actual New Cancer-Causing Hydrazines, Hydrazides and Hydrazones." *Journal of Cancer Research and Clinical Oncology*, vol. 97, no. 2, 1980, pp. 97–108.

11. Fletcher, Dean. "Do Reheated Frying Fats Contain Carcinogens?" *Journal of the American Medical Association*, January 30, 1978, p. 441.

Chapter 9: Diabetes

1. Holman, R. R. et al. "Prevention of Deterioration of Renal and Sensory-Nerve Function by More Intensive Management of Insulin-Dependent Diabetic Patients." *Lancet*, January 29, 1983, pp. 204–205.

2. Lauritzen, T. et al. "Effect of 6 Months of Strict Metabolic Control on Eye and Kidney Function in Insulin-Dependent Diabetics with Background Retinopathy." *Lancet*, January 16, 1982, pp. 121–123.

3. Simpson, H. C. et al. "A High Carbohydrate Leguminous Fibre Diet Improves All Aspects of Diabetic Control." *Lancet*, January 3, 1981, pp. 1–5.

4. Jenkins, David J. "Diabetes and Hyperlipidemia: Dietary Implications of Treatment with Fiber." *Practical Cardiology*, vol. 6, no. 11, 1980, pp. 123–134.

5. Funk, C., and Corbitt, H. B. "The Presence of a Blood-Sugar Reducing Substance in Yeast." *Proceedings of the Society for Experimental Biology and Medicine*, vol. 20, no. 207, 1923, pp. 422–423.

6. Offenbacher, Esther G., and Pi-Sunyer, F. X. "Beneficial Effect of Chromium-rich Yeast on Glucose Tolerance and Blood Lipids in Elderly Subjects." *Diabetes*, November, 1980, pp. 919–925.

7. Stout, Robert W. "The Relationship of Abnormal Circulating Insulin Levels to Atherosclerosis." *Atherosclerosis*, vol. 27, no. 1, 1977, pp. 1–13.

8. Davis, R. E.; Calder, J. S.; and Curnow, D. H. "Serum Pyridoxal and Folate Concentrations in Diabetics." *Pathology*, April, 1976, pp. 151–156.

9. Dubuc, D. "A Propos de la Vitamine B₆ (ou pyridoxine) et de l'Utilité de l'Observation en Médecine. *Journal de Médecine De Bordeaux*, vol. 138, 1961, pp. 881–882.

10. Schlütz, Von Georg Otto. "Über das Vorkommen von Pyridoxin—Mangeldiabetes in Nord-Sumatra." *Int. Z. Vitaminforsch*, vol. 33, 1963, pp. 150–153.

11. Spellacy, W. N.; Buhi, W. C.; and Birk, S. A. "The Effects of Vitamin B₆ on Carbohydrate Metabolism in Women Taking Steroid Contraceptives: Preliminary Report." *Contraception*, October, 1972, pp. 265–273.

12. Adams, P. W. et al. "Influence of Oral Contraceptives, Pyridoxine (vitamin B₆), and Tryptophan on Carbohydrate Metabolism." *Lancet*, April 10, 1976, pp. 759–764.

13. Rao, R. H., Vigg, B. L.; and Rao, K. S. "Failure of Pyridoxine to Improve Glucose Tolerance in Diabetics." *Journal of Clinical Endocrinology and Metabolism*, vol. 50, no. 1, 1980, pp. 198–200.

14. Kotake, Y., and Murakami, E. "A Possible Diabetogenic Role for Tryptophan Metabolites and Effects of Xanthurenic Acid on Insulin." *American Journal of Clinical Nutrition*, July, 1971, pp. 826–829.

15. McCann, V. J., and Davis, R. E. "Serum Pyridoxal Concentrations in Patients with Diabetic Neuropathy." *Australian and New Zealand Journal of Medicine*, June, 1978, pp. 259–261.

16. Jones, Charles, L., and Gonzalez, V. "Pyridoxine Deficiency: A New Factor in Diabetic Neuropathy." *Journal of the American Podiatry Association*, September, 1978, pp. 646–653.

17. Levin, Ellis R. et al. "The Influence of Pyridoxine in Diabetic Peripheral Neuropathy." *Diabetes Care*, vol. 4, no. 6, 1981, pp. 606–609.

18. Sancetta, Salvatore M.; Ayres, Perry R.; and Scott, Roy W. "The Use of Vitamin B_{12} in the Management of the Neurological Manifestations of Diabetes Mellitus with Notes on the Administration of Massive Doses." *Annals of Internal Medicine*, vol. 35, November, 1951, pp. 1028–1048.

19. Khan, M. A.; Wakefield, G. S.; and Pugh, D. W. "Vitamin B_{12} Deficiency and Diabetic Neuropathy," *Lancet*, October 11, 1969, pp. 768–769.

20. Davis R. E. et al. "The Association of Bacteriuria and Reduced Serum Pyridoxal Concentrations in Patients with Diabetes Mellitus." *Pathology*, July, 1981, pp. 587–591.

Chapter 10: Systemic Lupus Erythematosus

1. Dubois, Edmund L., ed. "The Clinical Picture of Systemic Lupus Erythematosus." In *Lupus Erythematosus*. 2d ed. University of Southern California Press, 1976, pp. 232–379.

2. DuBois, Edmund L., ed. "Chapter 15 Supplement: Results of Steroid Therapy in Systemic Lupus Erythematosus." In *Lupus Erythematosus*. 2d ed. University of Southern California Press, 1976, pp. 628–632.

3. Alberti-Flor, Juan J. "Chlorpromazine-induced Lupus-like Illness." *American Family Physician*, April, 1983, pp. 151–152.

4. Rumsby, P. C., and Shepherd, D. M. "Effect of Penicillamine, Hydrallazine, and Phenelzine on the Function of Pyridoxal-5'-Phosphate." *British Journal of Pharmacology*, July, 1979, pp. 453P–454P.

5. Swartz, Conrad. "Lupus-like Reaction to Phenelzine." *Journal of the American Medical Association*, June 23, 1978, p. 2693.

6. Lumeng, Lawrence; Cleary, Robert E.; and Li, Ting-Kai. "Effect of Oral Contraceptives on the Plasma Concentration of Pyridoxal Phosphate." *American Journal of Clinical Nutrition*, April, 1974, pp. 326–333.

7. Biehl, J. Park, and Vilter, Richard W. "Effects of Isoniazid on Pyridoxine Metabolism." *Journal of the American Medical Association*, December 25, 1954, pp. 1549–1552.

8. Zurier, Robert B. et al. "Prostaglandin E1 Treatment of NZB/NZW Mice." *Arthritis and Rheumatism*, March, 1977, pp. 723–728.

9. Horrobin, David F. "The Importance of Gamma-Linolenic Acid and Prostaglandin E1 in Human Nutrition and Medicine." *Journal of Holistic Medicine*, Fall/Winter, 1981, pp. 118–139.

10. Sagawa, Akira, and Abdou, Nabih I. "Suppressor-Cell Antibody in Systemic Lupus Erythematosus." *Journal of Clinical Investigation*, March, 1979, pp. 536–539.

11. Malinow, M. René; Bardana, Emil J., Jr.; and McLaughlin, Phyllis. "Systemic Lupus Erythematosus-like Syndrome in Monkeys Fed Alfalfa Sprouts: Role of a Nonprotein Amino Acid." *Science*, April 23, 1982, pp. 415–417.

12. Rosenthal, Gerald A. "A Mechanism of L-Canaline Toxicity." *European Journal of Biochemistry*, February, 1981, pp. 301–304.

13. Wright, Jonathan V. Personal Communication.

Chapter 11: Kidney Stones

1. Ettinger, Bruce. "Calcium Oxalate Stones: A Reappraisal of Their Work-Up and Prevention." *Medical Times*, November, 1981, pp. 20s–28s.

2. Johansson, G. et al. "Effects of Magnesium Hydroxide in Renal Stone Disease." *Journal of the American College of Nutrition*, vol. 1, no. 2, 1982, pp. 179–185.

3. Robertson, W. G., and Pencock, M. "The Cause of Idiopathic Calcium Stone Disease: Hypercalciuria or Hyperoxaluria?" *Nephron*, vol. 26, no. 3, 1980, pp. 105–110.

4. Shah, P. J.; Williams, Gordon; and Green, N. A. "Idiopathic Hypercalciuria: Its Control with Unprocessed Bran." *British Journal of Urology*, December, 1980, pp. 426–429.

5. Thom, J. A. et al. "The Influence of Refined Carbohydrate on Urinary Calcium Excretion." *British Journal of Urology*, December, 1978, pp. 459–464.

6. Robertson, W. G. et al. "Should Recurrent Calcium Oxalate Stone Formers Become Vegetarians?" *British Journal of Urology*, December, 1979, pp. 427–431.

7. Ringsdorf, W. M., Jr., and Cheraskin, E. "Nutritional Aspects of Urolithiasis." *Southern Medical Journal*, January, 1981, pp. 41–43, 46.

8. Gershoff, Stanley N. et al. "Vitamin B$_6$ Deficiency and Oxalate Nephrocalcinosis in the Cat." *American Journal of Medicine*, July, 1959, pp. 72–80.

9. Murphy, M. S. R. et al. "Effect of Pyridoxine Supplementation on Recurrent Stone Formers." *International Journal of Clinical Pharmacology, Therapy and Toxicology*, vol. 20, no. 9, 1982, pp. 434–437.

10. Gershoff, Stanley N., and Prien, Edwin L. "Effect of Daily MgO and Vitamin B$_6$ Administration to Patients with Recurring Calcium Oxalate Kidney Stones." *American Journal of Clinical Nutrition*, May, 1967, pp. 393–399.

11. Prien, Edwin L., Sr., and Gershoff, Stanley F. "Magnesium Oxide—Pyridoxine Therapy for Recurrent Calcium Oxalate Calculi." *Journal of Urology*, October, 1974, pp. 509–512.

12. Azoury, R. et al. "May Enzyme Activity in Urine Play a Role in Kidney Stone Formation?" *Urological Research*, vol. 10, no. 4, 1982, pp. 185–189.

13. McGeown, Mary G. "The Urinary Excretion of Amino Acids in Calculus Patients." *Clinical Science*, May, 1959, pp. 185–194.

14. Azoury, R. et al. "Retardation of Calcium Oxalate Precipitation by Glutamic-Oxalacetic-Transaminase Activity." *Urological Research*, vol. 10, no. 4, 1982, pp. 169–172.

15. Will, Eric J., and Bijvoet, Olav L. M. "Primary Oxalosis: Clinical and Biochemical Response to High-Dose Pyridoxine Therapy." *Metabolism*, May, 1979, pp. 542–548.

16. Balcke, P. et al. "Effect of Vitamin B$_6$ Administration on Elevated Plasma Oxalic Acid Levels in Haemodialysed Patients." *European Journal of Clinical Investigation*, December, 1982, pp. 481–483.

17. Wright, Jonathan V. "High-Dose Vitamin C and Kidney Stones." In *Dr. Wright's Book of Nutritional Therapy*. Rodale Press, 1979, pp. 272–277.

Chapter 12: Arthritis and Muscle Spasm

1. Ellis, John M., and Presley, James. *Vitamin B$_6$: The Doctor's Report*. Harper and Row, 1973, pp. 39–73.

2. Ellis, John M. et al. "Survey and New Data on Treatment with Pyridoxine of Patients Having a Clinical Syndrome Including the Carpal

Tunnel and Other Defects." *Research Communications in Chemical Pathology and Pharmacology*, May, 1977, pp. 165–177.

3. Turlapaty, Prasad D., and Altura, Burton M. "Magnesium Deficiency Produces Spasms of Coronary Arteries: Relationship to Etiology of Sudden Death Ischemic Heart Disease." *Science*, April, 1980, pp. 198–200.

Chapter 13: Carpal Tunnel Syndrome

1. Sandzen, Sigurd C., Jr. "Carpal Tunnel Syndrome." *American Family Physician*, November, 1981, pp. 190–204.

2. Ellis, John M., and Presley, James. "Rheumatism and the Carpal Tunnel Syndrome." In *Vitamin B₆: The Doctor's Report*. Harper and Row, 1973, pp. 57–73.

3. Phalen, George S., "The Birth of a Syndrome or Carpal Tunnel Revisited." *Journal of Hand Surgery*, vol. 6, 1981, pp. 109–110.

4. Ellis, John M. et al. "Survey and New Data on Treatment with Pyridoxine of Patients Having a Clinical Syndrome Including the Carpal Tunnel and Other Defects." *Research Communications in Chemical Pathology and Pharmacology*, May, 1977, pp. 165–177.

5. Ellis, John M. et al. "Response of Vitamin B₆ Deficiency and the Carpal Tunnel Syndrome to Pyridoxine." *Proceedings of the National Academy of Sciences*, December, 1982, pp. 7494–7498.

Chapter 14: Anemia

1. Wintrobe, Maxwell M. et al., eds. "Disorders of the Hematopoietic System." In *Harrison's Principles of Internal Medicine*. 7th ed. McGraw-Hill Book Company, 1974, pp. 1584–1585.

2. Beeson, Paul B.; McDermott, Walsh; and Wyngaarden, James B., eds. "Hematologic and Hematopoietic Diseases: Sideroblastic Anemia. In *Textbook of Medicine/Cecil*. 15th ed. W. B. Saunders Company, 1979, pp. 1740–1741.

3. Hines, John D., and Love, David. "Abnormal Vitamin B₆ Metabolism in Sideroblastic Anemia: Effect of Pyridoxal Phosphate (PLP) Therapy." *Clinical Research*, vol. 23, 1975, p. 403A.

4. Haden, Halcott T. "Pyridoxine-Responsive Sideroblastic Anemia Due to Antituberculous Drugs." *Archives of Internal Medicine*, November, 1967, pp. 602–606.

5. Rojer, Robert A.; Mulder, Nanno H.; and Nieweg, Hendrik O. "Response to Pyridoxine Hydrochloride in Refractory Anemia Due to Myelofibrosis." *American Journal of Medicine*, October, 1978, pp. 655–660.

6. Tant, Darryl. "Megaloblastic Anaemia Due to Pyridoxine Deficiency Associated with Prolonged Ingestion of an Oestrogen-Containing Oral Contraceptive." *British Medical Journal*, October 23, 1976, pp. 979–980.

7. Lutz, Howard. "Shotgun Hematinic Therapy." *Archives of Internal Medicine*, April, 1979, pp. 489–490.

8. Horrigan, Daniel L. "Pyridoxine-Responsive Anemia: Influence of Tryptophan on Pyridoxine Responsiveness." *Blood*, August, 1973, pp. 187–193.

Chapter 15: Alcoholism

1. Saxe, Leonard et al. "Summary." In *Health Technology Case Study 22: The Effectiveness and Costs of Alcoholism Treatment*. U.S. Government Printing Office, p. 1.

2. Bonjour, J. P. "Vitamins and Alcoholism: III. Vitamin B_6." *International Journal for Vitamin and Nutrition Research*, March 5, 1980, pp. 215–230.

3. Beeson, Paul B.; McDermott, Walsh; and Wyngaarden, James B., eds. "Hematologic and Hematopoietic Diseases: Sideroblastic Anemia." *Textbook of Medicine/Cecil*. 15th ed. W. B. Saunders Company, 1979, pp. 1740–1741.

4. Wordsworth, V. P. "Intravenous Detoxication of Drunkenness." *British Medical Journal*, April 25, 1953, p. 935.

5. Pullar-Strecker, H. "Intravenous Detoxication of Drunkenness." *British Medical Journal*, April 25, 1953, p. 935.

6. "A Note on Vitamin B_6, with Reference to Its Use in the Intravenous Detoxication of Drunkenness." *Quarterly Journal of Studies on Alcohol*, vol. 15, 1954, p. 348.

7. Small, M. D. et al. "The Effect of Pyridoxine Hydrochloride in Acute Alcoholic Intoxication." *Journal of Laboratory and Clinical Medicine*, July, 1955, pp. 12–20.

8. Palmer, Edwin J. "Pyridoxine Hydrochloride in the Treatment of Acute Alcoholism and Delirium Tremens." *Virginia Medical Monthly,* January, 1955, pp. 15–16.

9. Atkinson, Gerald W., and Kappes, William C. "Pyridoxine (Vitamin B₆) in Alcoholism." *Virginia Medical Monthly,* September, 1956, pp. 391–393.

10. Lim, Pin, and Jacob, Edward. "Magnesium Status of Alcoholic Patients." *Metabolism,* November, 1972, pp. 1045–1051.

11. Flink, Edmund B. et al. "Magnesium Deficiency After Prolonged Parenteral Fluid Administration and After Chronic Alcoholism Complicated by Delirium Tremens." *Journal of Laboratory and Clinical Medicine,* February, 1954, pp. 169–183.

12. Kakuma, Shinichi et al. "Protection of Pyridoxal 5'-Phosphate Against Toxicity of Acetaldehyde to Hepatocytes." *Proceedings of the Society for Experimental Biology and Medicine,* December, 1981, pp. 325–329.

Chapter 16: Tooth Decay

1. Newbrun, Ernest. "Dietary Carbohydrates: Their Role in Cariogenicity." *Medical Clinics of North America,* September, 1979, pp. 1069–1086.

2. Pagniez, P., and de Gennes, L. "Urticaria and Mastication." Abstracted in *Journal of the American Medical Association,* vol. 76, 1921, p. 1801.

3. Hillman, Robert W. "Effect of Vitamin B₆ on Dental Caries in Man." *Vitamins and Hormones,* vol. 22, 1964, pp. 695–704.

4. Palazzo, Augstine; Cobe, Herbert M.; and Ploumis, Emanuel. "The Effect of Pyridoxine Supplements on the Oral Microbial Populations." *New York State Dental Journal,* August-September, 1959, pp. 303–307.

5. Strean, Lyon P. "The Importance of Pyridoxine in Effecting a Change in the Microflora of the Mouth and Intestines." *New York State Dental Journal,* February, 1957, pp. 85–87.

6. Strean, L. P.; Gilfillan, Elizabeth W.; and Emerson, Gladys A. "Suppressive Effect of Pyridoxine as Dietary Supplement on Dental Caries in Syrian Hamster." *New York State Dental Journal,* August-September, 1956, pp. 325–327.

7. Strean, Lyon P. et al. "The Importance of Pyridoxine in the Suppression of Dental Caries in School Children and Hamsters." *New York State Dental Journal*, March, 1958, pp. 133–137.

8. Cohen, Abram, and Rubin, Carl. "Pyridoxine Supplementation in the Suppression of Dental Caries." *Bulletin of the Philadelphia County Dental Society*, vol. 22, 1958, pp. 84–86.

9. Hillman, Robert W.; Cabaud, Philip G.; and Schenone, Roger A. "The Effects of Pyridoxine Supplements on the Dental Caries Experience of Pregnant Women." *American Journal of Clinical Nutrition*, June, 1962, pp. 512–515.

Chapter 17: Chinese Restaurant Syndrome

1. Swan, Geraldine, F. "Management of Monosodium Glutamate Toxicity." *Journal of Asthma*, vol. 19, no. 2, 1982, pp. 105–110.

2. Schaumburg, Herbert H. et al. "Monosodium L-Glutamate: Its Pharmacology and Role in Chinese Restaurant Syndrome." *Science*, February 21, 1969, pp. 826–828.

3. Reif-Lehrer, Liane. "Possible Significance of Adverse Reactions to Glutamate in Humans." *Federation Proceedings*, September, 1976, pp. 2205–2212.

4. Ambos, Marjorie et al. "Sin Cib-Syn: Accent on Glutamate." *New England Journal of Medicine*, July 11, 1968, p. 105.

5. Neumann, Hans H. "Soup? It May Be Hazardous to Your Health." *American Heart Journal*, August, 1976, p. 266.

6. Reif-Lehrer, Liane, and Stemmerman, M. G. "Monosodium Glutamate Intolerance in Children." *New England Journal of Medicine*, December 4, 1975, p. 1204.

7. Rubini, M. E. "The Many-Faceted Mystique of Monosodium Glutamate." *American Journal of Clinical Nutrition*, February, 1971, pp. 169–171.

8. Zimmerman, Frederic T., and Burgemeister, Bessie B. "The Effect of Glutamic Acid on Borderline and High-Grade Defective Intelligence." *New York State Journal of Medicine*, March 15, 1950, pp. 693–697.

9. Price, J. C.; Waelsch, H.; and Putnam, T. J. "dl-Glutamic Acid Hydrochloride in Treatment of Petit Mal and Psychomotor Seizures."

Journal of the American Medical Association, August 21, 1943, pp. 1153–1156.

10. Shay, Harry, and Gershon-Cohen, J. "A Comparison of the Effectiveness of Glutamic Acid Hydrochloride and Dilute Hydrochloric Acid as the Replacement Therapy in Anacidity Measured by Fractional Gastric Acid Titration and Hydrogen-Ion Concentration Curves." *Annals of Internal Medicine*, vol. 9, 1936, pp. 1628–1638.

11. Schaumburg, Herbert H., and Byck, Robert. "Sin Cib-Syn: Accent on Glutamate." *New England Journal of Medicine*, July 11, 1968, p. 105.

12. "Pyridoxine Nutriture and Monosodium Glutamate Utilization by Rats." *Nutrition Reviews*, February 1973, pp. 70–71.

13. Wen, Chi-Pang, and Gershoff, Stanley, N. "Effects of Dietary Vitamin B_6 on the Utilization of Monosodium Glutamate by Rats." *Journal of Nutrition*, July, 1972, pp. 835–840.

14. Folkers, Karl et al. "Biochemical Evidence for a Deficiency of Vitamin B_6 in Subjects Reacting to Monosodium Glutamate by the Chinese Restaurant Syndrome." *Biochemical and Biophysical Research Communications*, June 16, 1981, pp. 972–977.

15. Dickey, Lawrence D., ed. "The Role of Specific Sugars." In *Clinical Ecology*. Charles C. Thomas, 1976, pp. 310–333.

Chapter 18: Asthma

1. Collipp, Platon J. et al. "Pyridoxine Treatment of Childhood Bronchial Asthma." *Annals of Allergy*, August, 1975, pp. 93–97.

Chapter 19: Other Ailments

1. Annand, J. C. "Pyridoxine and Magnesium in the Treatment of Shock." *Lancet*, August 17, 1957, pp. 340–341.

2. Rosenbaum, Edward E.; Portis, Sidney; and Soskin, Samuel. "The Relief of Muscular Weakness by Pyridoxine Hydrochloride." *Journal of Laboratory and Clinical Medicine*, vol. 27, 1941, pp. 763–770.

3. Antopol, William, and Schotland, Clement E. "The Use of Vitamin B_6 in Pseudohypertrophic Muscular Dystrophy." *Journal of the American Medical Association*, March 23, 1940, pp. 1058–1059.

4. Lewy, Alfred, and Fox, Noah. "Clinical Notes; New Instruments and Technics: Pyridoxine (B₆) Used in the Treatment of Vertigo." *Archives of Otolaryngology*, November, 1947, pp. 681–683.

5. Sanderson, C. R., and Davis, R. E. "Serum Pyridoxal in Active Peptic Ulceration. *Gut*, March, 1975, pp. 177–180.

6. Lindenbaum, Ella S., and Mueller, Joseph J. "Effects of Pyridoxine on Mice After Immobilization Stress." *Nutrition and Metabolism*, vol. 17, no. 6, 1974, pp. 368–374.

7. Jolliffe, Norman; Rosenblum, Louis A.; and Sawhill, John. "The Effects of Pyridoxine (Vitamin B₆) on Persistent Adolescent Acne." *Journal of Investigative Dermatology*, August, 1942, pp. 143–148.

8. Snider, B. Leonard, and Dieteman, David F. "Pyridoxine Therapy for Premenstrual Acne Flare." *Archives of Dermatology*, July, 1974, pp. 130–131.

9. Dorsey, Jodee L.; DeBruyne, Linda K.; and Rady, Sharon J. "The Effect of Vitamin B₆ Therapy on Premenstrual Acne and Tension." *Federation Proceedings*, vol. 42, no. 3, 1983, p. 556.

10. György, Paul. "Dietary Treatment of Scaly Desquamative Dermatoses of the Seborrheic Type." *Archives of Dermatology and Syphilology*, February, 1941, pp. 230–247.

11. Silbernagel, Wynne M., and Burt, Olan P. "Effects of Pyridoxine on Nausea and Vomiting of Pregnancy." *Ohio State Medical Journal*, December, 1943, pp. 1113–1114.

12. Wright, Carroll S.; Samitz, M. H.; and Brown, Herman. "Vitamin B₆ (Pyridoxine) in Dermatology." *Archives of Dermatology and Syphilology*, May, 1943, pp. 651–653.

13. Schreiner, A. William; Rockwell, Evelyn; and Vilter, Richard W. "Preliminary and Short Reports: A Local Defect in the Metabolism of Pyridoxine in the Skin of Persons with Seborrheic Dermatitis of the 'Sicca' Type." *Journal of Investigative Dermatology*, August, 1952, pp. 95–96.

14. Nisenson, Aaron. "Seborrheic Dermatitis of Infants and Leiner's Disease: A Biotin Deficiency." *Journal of Pediatrics*, vol. 51, 1957, pp. 537–548.

15. Mandel, Edward H. "New Treatment for Photosensitive Skin Eruptions: Results Obtained with Vitamin B$_6$." *New York State Journal of Medicine,* July 15, 1963, pp. 2097–2100.

16. Burkhart, Craig G. "Pyridoxine-Responsive Herpes Gestationis." *Archives of Dermatology,* August, 1982, p. 535.

17. Fosnaugh, Robert P.; Bryan, Henry G.; and Orders, Richard L. "Pyridoxine in the Treatment of Herpes Gestationis." *Archives of Dermatology,* July, 1961, pp. 140–145.

18. Coursin, David B. "Convulsive Seizures in Infants with Pyridoxine-Deficient Diet." *Journal of the American Medical Association,* January 30, 1954, pp. 406–408.

19. Bankier, A.; Turner, M.; and Hopkins, I. J. "Pyridoxine Dependent Seizures—A Wider Clinical Spectrum." *Archives of Disease in Childhood,* June, 1983, pp. 415–418.

20. Hansson, O., and Sillanpaa, M. "Pyridoxine and Serum Concentration of Phenytoin and Phenobarbitone." *Lancet,* January 31, 1976, p. 256.

21. Meller, Charlotte L. "Ten Cases of Paralysis Agitans Treated with Vitamin B$_6$." *Minnesota Medicine,* January, 1942, pp. 22–24.

22. Baker, A. B. "Treatment of Paralysis Agitans with Vitamin B$_6$ (Pyridoxine Hydrochloride)." *Journal of the American Medical Association,* May 31, 1941, pp. 2484–2487.

23. Zeligs, Meyer A. "Use of Pyridoxine Hydrochloride (Vitamin B$_6$) in Parkinsonism." *Journal of the American Medical Association,* May 10, 1941, pp. 2148–2149.

24. Barker, W. Halsey et al. "Failure of Pyridoxine (Vitamin B$_6$) to Modify the Parkinsonian Syndrome." *Bulletin of the Johns Hopkins Hospital,* September, 1941, pp. 266–275.

25. Leon, Arthur S, et al. "Pyridoxine Antagonism of Levodopa in Parkinsonism." *Journal of the American Medical Association,* December 27, 1971, pp. 1924–1927.

26. Mars, Harold. "Levodopa, Carbidopa, and Pyridoxine in Parkinson Disease: Metabolic Interactions." *Archives of Neurology,* June, 1974, pp. 444–447.

27. Airoldi, Luisa et al. "Effect of Pyridoxine on the Depletion of Tissue Pyridoxal Phosphate by Carbidopa." *Metabolism*, July, 1978, pp. 771–779.

28. Golden, Richard L. et al. "Levodopa, Pyridoxine, and the Burning Feet Syndrome," *Journal of the American Medical Association*, July 27, 1970, p. 628.

29. Kierska, D.; Sasiak, K.; and Maśliński, Cz. "Phosphopyridoxal Cyclic Compounds with Histamine and Histidine. 6: The Formation of Phosphopyridoxal Cyclic Compounds with Histamine and Histidine in the Presence of Biological Material." *Agents and Actions*, October, 1978, pp. 470–473.

30. Alvarez, Ricardo G., and Mesa, Milagros G. "Ascorbic Acid and Pyridoxine in Experimental Anaphylaxis." *Agents and Actions*, April, 1981, pp. 89–93.

31. Galeotti Flori, A., and Donatelli, L. "Sulle Proprietà Antiallergiche Della Vitamina B_6 [Antiallergic properties of vitamin B_6]." *Nutrition Abstracts and Reviews*, October, 1950, p. 327.

32. van Bijsterveld, O. P. "Pyridoxine Deficiency and the Conjunctiva." *Ophthalmologica*, vol. 173, no. 3–4, 1976, pp. 334–339.

33. Horrobin, D. F.; Campbell, A.; and McEwen, C. G. "Treatment of the Sicca Syndrome and Sjögren's Syndrome with E.F.A., Pyridoxine, and Vitamin C." *Progress in Lipid Research*, vol. 20, 1981, pp. 253–254.

34. Campbell, A. J., and McEwan, G. C. "Treatment of Brittle Nails and Dry Eyes." *British Journal of Dermatology*, July, 1981, p. 113.

35. McKendry, Robert J. R. "Treatment of Sjögren's Syndrome with Essential Fatty Acids, Pyridoxine and Vitamin C." *Prostaglandins, Leukotrienes and Medicine*, April, 1982, pp. 403–408.

36. Reeves, Robert J. "Treatment of Roentgen Sickness with Oral Administration of Pyridoxine Hydrochloride (Vitamin B_6)." *Southern Medical Journal*, May, 1946, pp. 405–407.

37. Stoll, Basil A. "Radiation Sickness: An Analysis of Over 1,000 Controlled Drug Trials." *British Medical Journal*, August 25, 1962, pp. 507–510.

38. Shorvon, L. M. "A Further Survey of Radiation Sickness with Particular Reference to Its Treatment by Pyridoxine." *British Journal of Radiology*, January, 1949, pp. 49–55.

39. Johnson, Carol G.; Vilter, Carl F.; and Spies, Tom D. "Irradiation Sickness in Rats." *American Journal of Roentgenology*, November, 1946, pp. 631–639.

40. Godel, J. C. "Trial of Pyridoxine Therapy for Tetanus Neonatorum." *Journal of Infectious Diseases*, April, 1982, pp. 547–549.

Chapter 20: How to Use B₆ Safely

1. Brenner, Arnold. "The Effects of Megadoses of Selected B Complex Vitamins on Children with Hyperkinesis: Controlled Studies with Long-Term Follow-up." *Journal of Learning Disabilities*, May, 1982, pp. 258–264.

2. Schaumburg, Herbert et al. "Sensory Neuropathy from Pyridoxine Abuse." *New England Journal of Medicine*, August 25, 1983, pp. 445–448.

3. Wason, Suman; Lacouture, Peter G; and Lovejoy, Frederick H. "Single High-Dose Pyridoxine Treatment for Isoniazid Overdose." *Journal of the American Medical Association*, September 4, 1981, pp. 1102–1104.

4. Frimpter, George W.; Andelman, Robert J.; and George, Walter F. "Vitamin B₆-Dependency Syndromes: New Horizons in Nutrition." *American Journal of Clinical Nutrition*, June, 1969, pp. 794–805.

5. Lauersen, Neils H., and Graves, Zoe R. "A New Approach to Premenstrual Syndrome." *The Female Patient*, April, 1983, pp. 41–55.

6. Will, Eric J., and Bijvoet, Olav L. M. "Primary Oxalosis: Clinical and Biochemical Response to High-Dose Pyridoxine Therapy." *Metabolism*, May, 1979, pp. 542–548.

7. Schaeppi, U., and Krinke, G. "Pyridoxine Neuropathy: Correlation of Functional Tests and Neuropathology in Beagle Dogs Treated with Large Doses of Vitamin B₆." *Agents and Actions*, vol. 12, no. 4, 1982, pp. 575–582.

8. Unna, Klaus, and Clark, Josephine D. "Effect of Large Amounts of Single Vitamins of the B Group upon Rats Deficient in Other Vita-

mins." *American Journal of the Medical Sciences,* vol. 204, 1942, pp. 364–371.

9. Rimland, Bernard. "An Orthomolecular Study of Psychotic Children." *Journal of Orthomolecular Psychiatry,* vol. 3, no. 4, 1974, pp. 371–377.

10. Molimard, R. et al. "Impairment of Memorization by High Doses of Pyridoxine in Man." *Biomedicine,* May, 1980, pp. 88–92.

11. Driskell, Judy A., and Loker, Sevim F. "Behavioral Patterns of Female Rats Fed High Levels of Vitamin B_6." *Nutrition Reports International,* October, 1976, pp. 467–473

Chapter 22: B_6's Biochemistry in Action

1. "The Interrelationship between Riboflavin and Pyridoxine." *Nutrition Reviews,* vol. 35, no. 9, 1977, p. 237.

2. Middleton, Henry M. "Intestinal Absorption of Pyridoxal-5'-Phosphate: Disappearance from Perfused Segments of Rat Jejunum In Vivo." *Journal of Nutrition,* vol. 109, no. 6, 1979, pp. 975–981.

3. Horrobin, David F. "The Importance of Gamma-linolenic Acid and Prostaglandin E1 in Human Nutrition and Medicine." *Journal of Holistic Medicine,* vol. 3, no. 2, 1981, pp. 118–139.

4. Bird, Timothy A., and Levene, Charles I. "Lysyl Oxidase: Evidence that Pyridoxal Phosphate Is a Cofactor." *Biochemical and Biophysical Research Communications,* vol. 108, no. 3, 1982, pp. 1172–1180.

5. Evans, G. W. "Normal and Abnormal Zinc Absorption in Man and Animals: The Tryptophan Connection." *Nutrition Reviews,* vol. 38, no. 4, 1980, pp. 137–141.

6. Krieger, Ingeborg. "Picolinic Acid in the Treatment of Disorders Requiring Zinc Supplementation." *Nutrition Reviews,* vol. 38, no. 4, 1980, pp. 148–150.

7. Leuthauser, Susan W.; Oberley, Larry W.: and Oberley, Terry D. "Antitumor Activity of Picolinic Acid in CBA/J Mice." *Journal of the National Cancer Institute,* vol, 68, no. 1, 1982, pp. 123–126.

8. Young, Jerry M., Jr.; Dinning, James S.; and Day, Paul L. "Metabolic Interrelationships of Vitamins E and B_6." *Proceedings of the Society for Experimental Biology and Medicine,* vol. 89, 1955, pp. 216–217.

9. "Probe Nutrient Roles in Heart Diseases, Cancer and Ileitis." *Hospital Practice*, January, 1983, pp. 153–154.

10. Abraham, Guy E.; Schwartz, Ulf D.; and Lubran, Michael M. "Effect of Vitamin B$_6$ on Plasma and Red Blood Cell Magnesium Levels in Premenopausal Women." *Annals of Clinical and Laboratory Science*, vol. 11, no. 4, 1981, pp. 333–335.

FOOD SOURCES OF VITAMIN B$_6$

The table below lists a sampling of foods that are rich in vitamin B$_6$, arranged from highest to lowest B$_6$ content. The foods are presented in typical serving portions, with the amount of B$_6$ per portion given in milligrams. These amounts hold only for foods prepared as listed. Cooking, freezing and processing alter the vitamin content of raw foods, and this should be taken into account when estimating your own intake of vitamins from food.

Food	Portion	Vitamin B$_6$ (milligrams)
100% bran cereal	1 cup	2.1
40% bran flakes cereal	1 cup	0.80
Watermelon	1 slice	0.69
Banana	1	0.66
Salmon, raw	3 ounces	0.63

Continued

Sources: Adapted from

Pantothenic Acid, Vitamin B$_6$ and Vitamin B$_{12}$ in Foods, Home Economics Research Report No. 36, by Martha Louise Orr (Washington, D.C.: Agricultural Research Service, U.S. Department of Agriculture, 1969).

Nutritive Value of American Foods in Common Units, Agriculture Handbook No. 456, by Catherine F. Adams (Washington, D.C.: Agricultural Research Service, U.S. Department of Agriculture, 1975).

Composition of Foods: Fruits and Fruit Juices, Agriculture Handbook No. 8-9, by Consumer Nutrition Center (Washington, D.C.: Human Nutrition Information Service, U.S. Department of Agriculture, 1982).

Composition of Foods: Dairy and Egg Products, Agriculture Handbook No. 8-1, by Consumer and Food Economics Institute (Washington, D.C.: Agricultural Research Service, U.S. Department of Agriculture, 1976).

Composition of Foods: Breakfast Cereals, Agriculture Handbook No. 8-8, by Consumer Nutrition Center (Washington, D.C.: Human Nutrition Information Service, U.S. Department of Agriculture, 1982).

Composition of Foods: Soups, Sauces, and Gravies, Agriculture Handbook No. 8-6, by Consumer and Food Economics Institute (Washington, D.C.: Science and Education Administration, U.S. Department of Agriculture, 1980).

Composition of Foods: Poultry Products, Agriculture Handbook No. 8-5, by Consumer and Food Economics Institute (Washington, D.C.: Science and Education Administration, U.S. Department of Agriculture, 1979).

McCance and Widdowson's The Composition of Foods, by A. A. Paul and D. A. T. Southgate (New York: Elsevier/North-Holland Biomedical, 1978).

FOOD SOURCES OF VITAMIN B₆—*Continued*

Food	Portion	Vitamin B₆ (milligrams)
Chicken, light meat without skin	3 ounces	0.51
Tomato paste	½ cup	0.50
Chicken liver	3 ounces	0.49
Turkey, light meat without skin	3 ounces	0.48
Beef liver	3 ounces	0.47
Tomato juice	1 cup	0.47
Trout, Rainbow or Steelhead, raw	3 ounces	0.47
Mackerel, Atlantic, raw	3 ounces	0.45
Sunflower seeds	¼ cup	0.45
Granola cereal	1 cup	0.43
Soybeans, dry	¼ cup	0.43
Pork	3 ounces	0.40
Halibut, Atlantic or Pacific, raw	3 ounces	0.39
Sweet potato, raw	1 medium	0.39
Potato, raw	1 medium	0.38
Tuna, canned	3 ounces	0.36
Herring, Atlantic, raw	3 ounces	0.34
Turkey, dark meat without skin	3 ounces	0.32
Chicken, dark meat without skin	3 ounces	0.31
Broccoli, raw	1 medium stalk	0.29
Avocado	½	0.28
Brown rice, raw	¼ cup	0.28
Sirloin	3 ounces	0.28
Chick-peas, dried	¼ cup	0.27
Crab	3 ounces	0.26
Manhattan clam chowder	1 cup	0.26
Beef kidney	3 ounces	0.24
Pineapple juice	1 cup	0.24
Walnuts, English, chopped	¼ cup	0.22

Food	Portion	Vitamin B₆ (milligrams)
Veal	3 ounces	0.22
Ocean perch	3 ounces	0.21
Brewer's yeast	1 tablespoon	0.20
Cod, raw	3 ounces	0.20
Brussels sprouts, raw	4	0.19
Vegetable soup	1 cup	0.19
Filberts, shelled	¼ cup	0.18
Soybean flour, defatted	¼ cup	0.18
Lima beans, immature, cooked	½ cup	0.17
Chili beef soup	1 cup	0.16
Pomegranate	1 medium	0.16
Squash, winter, raw	½ cup	0.16
Cantaloupe	¼	0.15
Flounder, raw	3 ounces	0.15
Gazpacho soup	1 cup	0.15
Sardines, Atlantic, canned in oil	3 ounces	0.15
Sauerkraut	½ cup	0.15
Spinach, raw, chopped	1 cup	0.15
Buckwheat flour, dark	¼ cup	0.14
Mango	½	0.14
Peanuts, roasted, chopped	¼ cup	0.14
Brie	2 ounces	0.13
Camembert	2 ounces	0.13
Chestnuts, shelled	¼ cup	0.13
Corn, frozen, sweet, yellow, cut	½ cup	0.13
Cauliflower, raw, florets	½ cup	0.11
Figs	2 medium	0.11
Goat's milk	1 cup	0.11
Milk, lowfat	1 cup	0.11
Peanut butter	2 tablespoons	0.11
Prunes, dried	5	0.11
Yogurt, plain, lowfat	1 cup	0.11

Continued

FOOD SOURCES OF VITAMIN B₆—*Continued*

Food	Portion	Vitamin B₆ (milligrams)
Asparagus, raw	½ cup	0.10
Bulgur, dry	¼ cup	0.10
Collards, frozen, chopped	½ cup	0.10
Green pea soup	1 cup	0.10
Leeks	¼ cup	0.10
Milk, skim	1 cup	0.10
Orange juice	1 cup	0.10
Raisins	¼ cup	0.10
Rye flour, dark	¼ cup	0.10
Whole wheat flour	¼ cup	0.10
Black bean soup	1 cup	0.09
Blue cheese	2 ounces	0.09
Cabbage, red, raw, chopped	½ cup	0.09
Dates, dried	¼ cup	0.09
Shredded wheat cereal, large biscuit	1 cup	0.09
Milk, dry, nonfat, reconstituted	1 cup	0.08
Orange	1 medium	0.08
Apple	1 medium	0.07
Pineapple	1 slice	0.07
Cream of mushroom soup	1 cup	0.06
Egg, hard-cooked	1	0.06
Kale, raw	½ cup	0.06
Onions, raw	¼ cup	0.06
Oyster stew	1 cup	0.06
Turnips, raw	½ cup	0.06
Wheat germ, toasted	1 tablespoon	0.06
Chicken soup	1 cup	0.05
Oatmeal, cooked	1 cup	0.05
Pecans, shelled	¼ cup	0.05
Whole wheat bread	1 slice	0.05
Colby cheese	2 ounces	0.04
Eggplant, raw	½ cup	0.04
Mushrooms, raw	½ cup	0.04
Watercress, raw	¼ cup	0.04

FOOD SOURCES OF MAGNESIUM

Since magnesium works together with B$_6$ in the body and enhances the effectiveness of vitamin B$_6$, you may wish to estimate the amount of magnesium in your diet. This table lists a sampling of magnesium-rich foods in order of magnesium content.

Food	Portion	Magnesium (milligrams)
Soybeans, dried	¼ cup	138
Blackeye peas, dried	¼ cup	98
Almonds	¼ cup	96
Tofu (soybean curd)	3 ounces	95
Cashews	¼ cup	94
Peas, dried	¼ cup	90
Lima beans, large, dried	¼ cup	81
Brazil nuts	¼ cup	79
Pecans, halved	¼ cup	77
Soybean flour, defatted	¼ cup	77
Kidney beans, dried	¼ cup	75
Shredded wheat cereal, spoon size	1 cup	65
Peanuts, roasted, chopped	¼ cup	63
Filberts, shelled	¼ cup	62

Continued

Sources: Adapted from

Composition of Foods, Agriculture Handbook No. 8, by Bernice K. Watt and Annabel L. Merrill (Washington, D.C.: Agricultural Research Service, U.S. Department of Agriculture, 1975).

Nutritive Value of American Foods in Common Units, Agriculture Handbook No. 456, by Catherine F. Adams (Washington, D.C.: Agricultural Research Service, U.S. Department of Agriculture, 1975).

Composition of Foods: Dairy and Egg Products, Agriculture Handbook No. 8-1, by Consumer and Food Economics Institute (Washington, D.C.: Agricultural Research Service, U.S. Department of Agriculture, 1976).

Composition of Foods: Spices and Herbs, Agriculture Handbook No. 8-2, by Consumer and Food Economics Institute (Washington, D.C.: Agricultural Research Service, U.S. Department of Agriculture, 1977).

Composition of Foods: Poultry Products, Agriculture Handbook No. 8-5, by Consumer and Food Economics Institute (Washington, D.C.: Science and Education Administration, U.S. Department of Agriculture, 1979).

FOOD SOURCES OF MAGNESIUM—*Continued*

Food	Portion	Magnesium (milligrams)
Walnuts, black, chopped	¼ cup	60
Banana	1 medium	58
Beet greens, raw, chopped	1 cup	58
Avocado	½	56
Buckwheat flour, light	¼ cup	56
Oatmeal, cooked	1 cup	56
Peanut flour	¼ cup	54
Blackstrap molasses	1 tablespoon	52
Potato, raw	1 medium	51
Spinach, raw, chopped	1 cup	48
Yogurt, plain, skim milk	1 cup	47
Brown rice, cooked	¾ cup	42
Swiss chard, raw, chopped	1 cup	36
Whole wheat flour	¼ cup	34
Milk, whole	1 cup	33
Salmon, Sockeye, canned, drained	3 ounces	32
Collards, raw	1 cup	31
Yogurt, plain, whole milk	1 cup	29
Milk, skim	1 cup	28
Peanut butter	1 tablespoon	28
Chicken, light meat without skin	3 ounces	24
Turkey, light meat without skin	3 ounces	24
Wheat germ, toasted	1 tablespoon	23
Ground beef, lean	3 ounces	21
Turkey, dark meat without skin	3 ounces	21
Chicken, dark meat without skin	3 ounces	20
Swiss cheese	2 ounces	20
Rye flour, light	¼ cup	19
Brewer's yeast	1 tablespoon	18

Food	Portion	Magnesium (milligrams)
Chestnuts, shelled	¼ cup	17
Cheddar cheese	2 ounces	16
Wheat bran	1 tablespoon	15
Ricotta cheese	½ cup	14
Apricots, dried	3 medium	13
Barley, pearled, light	⅛ cup	9
Cottage cheese	½ cup	6
Egg, hard-cooked	1	6
Parmesan cheese, grated	1 tablespoon	3
Parsley, dried	1 teaspoon	1
Curry powder	⅛ teaspoon	0.63
Chili powder	⅛ teaspoon	0.50

Index

A

Acetaldehyde, affecting liver cells, 152
Acidosis
    in diabetes, 108
    isoniazid causing, 9
Acne, 175–76
    premenstrual, 33, 176
Agaritine, 15, 198
Aircraft fuel, exposure to, 8
Alcoholism, 148–52
    delirium tremens in, 150–51
    liver damage in, 152
    magnesium deficiency in, 151
    vitamin B_6 in, 149–52
        sobering effects of, 149
Alfalfa sprouts
    L-canavanine in, 15
    lupus from, 119
Allergy, 181–82
    and anaphylactic shock, 182
    to food
        and arthritis, 133
        and attention deficit disorder, 74,
            75
        chewing affecting, 153
        to corn and beets, 165, 166
        depression in, 66–68
        and migraine, 4
        and reactions to monosodium
            glutamate, 159–67
Almonds, magnesium in, 241
Amines in brain
    antidepressants affecting, 60–61
    in depression, 60
    imbalance of, 69
    orthomolecular therapy affecting, 62–63
    in premenstrual syndrome, 27–28
Amino acid therapy, 62, 63
Amitriptyline, 60
Anaphylactic shock, 182

Anecdotal information, in research studies,
    192, 196–97
Anemia, 144–47
    folate deficiency, 146
    iron deficiency, 145
    in myelofibrosis, 3, 146
    pernicious, 2
    sideroblastic, 145–46
        in alcoholism, 148
        pyridoxal phosphate in, 145–46
        tryptophan therapy in, 147
    symptoms of, 144
    vitamin B_6 in, 145–47
Angina pectoris, magnesium affecting, 98
Angiotoxins, 96
Anticonvulsants, interaction with vitamin
    B_6, 179
Antidepressants, 60–63
Antihistamines, 181
Antimetabolites of vitamin B_6, 6–15
    dangers of, 197–98
    and enzyme activity, 17–18
    lupus from, 117
Apgar score, 52–53
Appetite
    in depression, 66
    vitamin B_6 affecting, 40–41
Apples, vitamin B_6 in, 240
Apricots, magnesium in, 243
Arrhythmias, in reaction to monosodium
    glutamate, 160
Arthritis, 130–34
    diet in, 133, 137
    rheumatoid, penicillamine in, 11
    vitamin B_6-responsive, 131–34
Asparagus, vitamin B_6 in, 240
Asthma, 3, 168–72
    avoidance of attack triggers in, 169
    in childhood, 3, 169, 170–72
    drug therapy in, 170

Rodale Press, Inc., publishes PREVENTION®, the better health magazine.
For information on how to order your subscription,
write to PREVENTION®, Emmaus, PA 18049.